= STILLPOINT =
The Dance of Selfcaring, Selfhealing

A PLAYBOOK
FOR PEOPLE WHO DO CARING WORK

SHEILA K. COLLINS, PhD

TLC
PRODUCTIONS

Published by TLC Productions Inc.
1152 Country Club Lane
Fort Worth, Texas, 76112
(817) 654-9600 Fax (817) 654-2256

© Copyright 1992 by Sheila K. Collins

Book and Cover Design: Bill Maize and Tom Dawson, Duo Design Group, Inc., Fort Worth, Texas

Cover artwork from a limited edition etching by Valerie Kneeland, Austin, Texas, (512) 441-6843

© 1991 "In Harmony", Valerie Kneeland

The publisher makes no warranty of any kind, expressed or implied, with regard to the information provided in this book.

First Printing: July, 1992

Printed in the United States of America on recycled paper.

Publisher's Cataloging in Publication Data

Collins, Sheila Katherine, 1939-
Stillpoint: the dance of selfcaring, selfhealing: a playbook for people who do caring work/Sheila K. Collins.
p. cm.
Pre-assigned LCCN: 91-68151
Includes bibliographical references and index.
ISBN: 0-9631856-0-8

1. Health promotion. 2. Caregivers 3. Social workers. 4. Nurses. 5. Self-care, Health. I. Title.

RA427.8.C6 1992   613
                    QBI92-509

Poems by Ralph Caplan copyright Herman Miller. Used by permission of Ralph Caplan and Herman Miller.

Excerpt from "The Art of Conscious Celebration: A New Concept For Today's Leaders," by Cathy DeForest. copyright 1985, in *Transforming Leadership: From Vision To Results*, John Adams, editor, Miles River Press, Alexandria, VA. copyright 1986. reprinted by permission of Miles River Press.

Excerpt from "Burnt Norton" in *Four Quartets*, copyright 1943 by T.S. Eliot and renewed 1971 by Esme Valerie Eliot, reprinted by permission of Harcourt Brace Jovanovich, Inc.

Reprinted from *Black Elk Speaks*, by John G. Neihardt, by permission of University of Nebraska Press. Copyright 1932, 1959, 1972, by John G. Neihardt. Copyright © 1961 by the John G. Neihardt Trust.

Song "Let There be Peace On Earth", copyright 1955 by Jan-Lee Music, renewed 1983, Used by permission of Jill Jackson Miller, Jan-Lee Music.

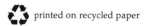 printed on recycled paper

To my teachers,
midwives, students, clients,
and dance instructors,
this book is dedicated

ACKNOWLEDGEMENTS

• •

Throughout the long, difficult process of birthing this book, many people provided invaluable assistance, encouragement, and inspiration. For their help with the stillborn version which preceded this present volume, I wish to thank Ilana Rubenfeld, Joan Lakin, Jim Collins, and Florence Korzinski, along with the 1984-1988 Rubenfeld Synergy training community who acted as fair witnesses to the emerging dancer struggling to become writer.

Colleagues in the helping professions who read the early drafts included Drs. Roy Martin, Jean Deschner, and Coleen Shannon, and student Laurel Chapet. I am grateful for their support and suggestions.

For help with the present version I wish to thank Ian Jackson who taught me some of what he knows about editing and shared his Breathplay and hypnosis work with me. Frances Townsend, a multi-talented woman, worked many hours with me on editing. She also shared with me some of her vast knowledge of nutrition and how to become selfcaring with food.

Special appreciation goes to the members of the Live Poets' Society: Dr. Gary and Victoria Campbell, Randall and Jyoti King, and Dr. Richard Citrin for forming a community around me when I was feeling most alone and teaching me that writing, too, can be a dance. Additional appreciation goes to Bertha Hendricks and Roy Martin for their help with the final editing phase.

I owe the deepest gratitude to my family, my husband Richard Citrin, and children, Corinne, Kevin, and Kenneth who supported me through the roller coaster rides of my career life and through many of the events on which this book is based.

Finally, and most especially, I wish to acknowledge and express my gratitude to two outstandingly powerful and brilliant women without whom this volume would never have been completed. Jyoti King and Rosa Marie Meile stayed beside me, editing, encouraging, and continuing to believe in me and this work even through the periods of my deepest discouragement. They, and many others un-named, have taught me the true meaning of partnership power.

OVERTURE

• •

It is said that we teach what we want to learn, and this seemed true as I set out on what has turned out to be a long journey to write this book about selfcaring. I believe now that the journey has been longer than I expected because I knew even less than I thought I did about how to be selfcaring. And I certainly didn't know that doing something in a selfcaring way would take so much longer.

Along the way in this "play within a play," as I attempted to use the book to develop my own selfcaring skills, I was met by challenging difficulties. In order to arrange time on my calendar for writing I needed to confront an old habit, organizing my life around the convenience of other people. I found it painfully difficult at times to tell clients, colleagues, and family members that I wouldn't be available when they wanted to see me.

Most of the people in my life stayed connected to me through the long book writing process. But I lost some relationships when I stopped playing by other people's rules.

I learned the connection between selfcaring and selfhealing when I sat down to write. Tuning in to myself in a selfcaring way to work on the book, I discovered my exhaustion. I realized I was overworking in order to get time to write. Then, before I could go forward in the preventive way of selfcaring, I had to back up and recover, caring enough about myself to do the hard work necessary for selfhealing.

I came to believe that the means used to achieve the book would be reflected in the book's final form. I felt , too, that the way I treated myself in the process would be a true measure of what I had learned. As I prepare to let go of these, by now, well worn pages, it is my hope that you, the reader, will use them gently, as an inspiration for your own self-discovery and recovery.

PLAYBILL

• •

STILLPOINT: The Dance of Selfcaring, Selfhealing

OVERTURE

ACT I: STEPS, TECHNIQUES, AND ESSENTIAL ELEMENTS

ACT II STAGE AND SETTING

ACT III: PRACTICE AND REHEARSAL

ACT IV : THE DANCE

PROLOGUE

●●●

The Dance of Selfcaring, Selfhealing

Caring for others is a hazardous occupation. Whether we work in a so-called "helping profession," hold a job in the service industry providing services to the public, or focus our caregiving on family and friends — the problem is the same. Those of us who care for others have trouble caring for ourselves.

PEOPLE WHO DO CARING WORK

In these days of computer technologists, financial planners, and wizards of leveraged buyouts and expansion, there is, in the work place as well as in the home place, a group of workers dedicated to the work of caring for others. Their number is growing, and their influence is beginning to be felt. As Newsweek has declared, "Greed Is Dead" for the 1990s, and more and more people are returning to jobs which involve service to others. In deep appreciation for the important contribution these peopleworkers make to the well-being of our world, they are coming to be known, respectfully, by the title CAREGIVER, which means *giver who cares.*

Traditionally, caregivers have been found in homes, schools, hospitals, and service organizations, both in salaried and volunteer positions. And they were most often female. However, recent changes in the economy that led to a decline in the number of manufacturing jobs have meant that many men, instead of "making widgets," now work at jobs tending to the needs of other people. This expansion in the service economy has created a whole new population of workers who engage in caring, helping, and other types of "hand-holding" with clients, patients, customers, and patrons. By the year 2000, if this trend continues, there will be nearly as many male caregivers as female. By all projections, a large number of people will be doing work which involves serving others. Due to the large number of people affected, it is fortunate that with the expanded meaning of the term *CAREGIVER* comes growing recognition of the caregivers' need and responsibility to give care to themselves. In order to preserve themselves as people capable of caring, caregivers are in need of the skills of selfcaring and selfhealing.

As a social work professor, I saw myself in my students and colleagues. We worked enthusiastically, helping and serving others. We continued caring for family and friends in our personal lives. But before long, rather than being people who had it all, we seemed more like people who do it all, with nothing left for ourselves.

And the same is true of the clients who have come to me for therapy through the years. Many are strong, generous people who have hurt themselves in the process of caring for others. They have taken care of family, friends, work, and community projects. They are in therapy quite a while before finally finding the courage to ask the question, "When is it my turn?" When I suggest that now is the best time to begin using some of their caring energy for themselves, they respond with blank expressions and admit, "I don't have the slightest idea how to do that!"

WHAT IS THE SITUATION?

As R.D.Laing, the iconoclastic British psychiatrist said, "Nobody in the situation knows what the situation is."[1] It's difficult to understand why selfcaring is so hard to do since we mention it to one another at practically every meeting. "Now, take care of yourself," a mother says to her grown daughter on their parting. "You take care now, you hear," one friend signals to another from across the street. It seems we're constantly making each other promise to take care of ourselves, reminding each other of the importance of selfcaring almost as often as we say good-by. In spite of these frequent reminders, we seem unaware of what the situation is, of what we are really up against.

Not knowing how to be selfcaring, we peopleworkers frequently injure ourselves. A leading researcher, Christina Maslach reported on her extensive research with nurses, teachers, social workers, police, and other peopleworkers in a book she titled, *Burnout -The Cost of Caring.*[2] The burnout Maslach documented amounts to emotional and physical overload leading to exhaustion. People suffering from burnout react to protect themselves by becoming detached, shutting down emotionally. Many report having feelings of wanting to be left alone and then feeling guilty for having such feelings. For some, a reduced sense of accomplishment occurs as they "go through the motions" without a real caring commitment. Others drop out of careers and relationships that they have invested years in building. From what we know about the stress of burnout, it is clear that strong, healthy people are especially vulnerable. Whether in our work or in our family lives, if we don't take care of ourselves we lose the ability to continue our lifestyle of caring connection to others.

So, what makes selfcaring so hard? How do we get so far off base that we need to take time out from our lives for recovery and healing? If we know how to care for others — children and jobs, friends, and good causes — what gets in the way of our including ourselves in all that caring energy?

Prior Injuries

One of the first problems in taking care of ourselves is what we have done to our bodies and what most people around us have done to theirs. After denying, ignoring, or perhaps even abusing our bodies, the distorted feedback we get interferes with our taking care of ourselves properly. Selfhealing then becomes a prerequisite to selfcaring, and selfcaring becomes a way to identify one's need to heal.

The roots of our disregard for ourselves run deep and wide. Caregiving historically has been women's work, and our masculine-focused tradition has devalued both women and the caring service they have provided. "I'm only a housewife" says as much about the culture as it does about the woman who describes herself in those terms.[3]

Whether male or female, many of us who do caring work as adults grew up playing the caretaking role in our families. In that situation, selfcaring meant taking care of the adults in our lives so they would be able to take care of us. We developed the habit of attempting to earn love by being good and doing good. Afraid to be called "selfish," we became "codependent," caring more for the people in a relationship or for the relationship itself than we cared for ourselves. It's easy to confuse selfcaring with being selfish. This sets the stage for overdoing our caring role and we become codependent workaholics, damaging ourselves as we serve others.

Becoming Selfcaring

In order to become selfcaring we must first reclaim and recondition our physical selves. We must rediscover our most neglected senses, our movement (kinesthetic) and touch (tactile) senses. These senses contain the information about how we are and what we need.

In order to become selfcaring we must become receptive to inner signals and give greater credence to our felt experience. Cultural habits of ignoring the intuitive, feminine way of knowing has us seeking perfection, operating from the abstract and theoretical while losing touch with ourselves and our human needs. Including the feminine means that we, both men and women, can seek completeness rather than perfection. Incorporating the intuitive feminine with the analytical masculine allows a creative synthesis. Then we can give attention to the context in which all this occurs.

Including the feminine gives us access to a caring ethic[4] which holds an important key to our selfcaring. Caring means being able to be receptive to the needs of others, to relate and respond to others and to the needs of the situation. But the feminine principle is inclusive, and it includes the needs of the caregiver as well.

Creative expression is a central human need often overlooked by those of us who care for others. Hans Selye,[5] the researcher who first identified stress, recommended creative expression of our real selves as the key to managing the stress of life. Viewing our life and work as continual opportunities to express ourselves creatively insures that we not bog down in routine, become overwhelmed by criticism, or take ourselves too seriously.

As I involved myself as a teacher and therapist in learning and teaching about selfcaring, I found myself drawing on my background as a dancer. Dancing has been a significant part of my life since childhood. I always knew that dancing was a way for me to take care of myself. As one of my dance teachers used to say, "Dancing doesn't take energy, it makes energy!" I didn't understand the reasons why dancing worked in this way, but even my own children, when they were young, noticed the connection between dancing and my ability to cope. When they saw me losing patience with them, they would suggest, "Don't you think it's time for you to take a dancing class, Mom?"

After a career as a dancer I entered the academic world where I was continually sensitive to the gaps and omissions in what was officially considered knowledge. Later, as a professor, I was criticized for my inclusion of physical aspects of the self in social work courses. My methods were labeled "touchy-feelie," and were considered offensive — a threat to true intellectual pursuit. I felt a bit like the child in the fairy tale "The Emperor's New Clothes" who informed the emperor of his nakedness, an obvious truth no one wanted to hear. In my case, I seemed to be continually reminding people of truths they were trying to forget, namely that there were physical bodies beneath those academic robes.

As a dancer, I have tremendous respect for the importance of technique. Technique builds the strength and skill to perform a great variety of movements while relating to other dancers and the audience. But a dancer's technique is only a vehicle for the creative expression of human experience including personal, emotional, and communal realities.

The dance of caring work is more than techniques, more than action steps. There are movements in which one expresses oneself, and pauses, and transitions of relating and responding to another. And most of all there is, for the caregiver as for the dancer, the use of one's physical self as the stuff of which the dance is made.

BODY/MIND CONNECTION

This book approaches selfcaring and selfhealing from the perspective of our psychobiology. Scientists are learning more each day about the effect of mental attitudes, emotions, and personality habits on body functioning. As Bernie Seigel demonstrates in *Love, Medicine and Miracles*,[6] when patients begin dealing with mental, emotional, and spiritual aspects of themselves, their recovery from serious illness is greatly enhanced.

This book focuses on the other side of that two way reciprocal connection, ways to change the body in order to affect our mental, emotional, and spiritual dimensions. The reciprocal communication which begins with the body is less familiar to most people than the other way around. It took a Shakespearean actor, F. M. Alexander, to discover that a physical symptom, laryngitis, could be caused by incorrect posture and what he called "the misuse of the self."[7]

Another recent contributor to information about our psychophysical nature is Moshe Feldenkrais, an Israeli physicist. Feldenkrais set out to heal himself from a karate injury and wound up mapping the central nervous system. He discovered that by using non-habitual movements done passively or slowly, in a state of relaxation, the brain is stimulated and the mind and body become more flexible.[8]

Ilana Rubenfeld, as a music conductor, developed chronic pain in her shoulder. In the search for her own healing she became an Alexander teacher (a system of body reeducation) and a student of both Fritz Perls (father of gestalt therapy) and Moshe Feldenkrais (Israeli master of movement education). Rubenfeld created a body-oriented psychotherapy, the Rubenfeld Synergy Method,[9] a synthesis of these methods. She added music, hypnosis and her own artistic expression of humor. While I was her student, her strong emphasis on selfcare sparked my interest in selfcaring and selfhealing.

Building on the work of these illustrious pioneers and manifested in the expression which is this book, my contribution as a dancer, social worker, and teacher is to teach caregivers how to dance the dance of selfcaring, selfhealing.

THE BENEFITS

As you learn more about your psychophysical self and the steps in the dance of selfcaring/selfhealing you will:

- Find and communicate with the parts of yourself that need your caring;
- Identify the elements missing in your selfcaring lifestyle;
- Increase your understanding of yourself as a strong, yet vulnerable living system;
- Learn ways to recondition your body's response to threat
- Learn selfcaring skills to take care of yourself while you are involved in caring for others in your family life;
- Learn to alter your work environment to support selfcaring for yourself and the others people who spend time there;
- Discover the use of creative expressions such as movement, music, and dance to release tension and generate positive energy;
- Explore humor as a tool of creative expression, to defuse or reframe difficult situations;
- Apply your creative and artistic talents in making your own healing rituals following the model provided.

GUIDE TO USING THIS BOOK

Selfcaring and selfhealing require moving beyond our logical, intellectual minds into the *kinesthetic, feminine,* and *creative* parts of ourselves. Throughout this book you will encounter these three terms representing aspects of ourselves often overlooked in our scientifically-oriented culture. The **kinesthetic** senses give us information about ourselves and the world through touch and internal and external sensations of our body. In our culture animals and young children are better at relying on these senses than adults whose education has stifled their ability to use them. The term **feminine** refers to the cluster of human qualities and abilities which exist in both men and women, but which have been historically assigned to women. Selfcaring and selfhealing for both men and women requires respecting and reclaiming these important human qualities. We explore **creativity** because many adults in our culture have become convinced that without special talent or expert training they cannot consider themselves creative or exercise this aspect of themselves.

This book is organized so as to encourage you, the reader, to explore and learn from your own as well as other people's experiences.

Since stories are a powerful way to learn what can be at times, mysterious principles, I have constructed stories from the experiences of many people I have worked with these past twenty years. To protect their privacy I have altered identifying information and sometimes combined experiences of more than one person into a single story. It is my hope that you will recognize yourself, as I did, in the people and situations illustrated.

Act One defines selfcare and its connection to selfhealing. We meet a pair of fanciful characters who help us better understand the scientific information about how one's body and mind work together. Five selfcaring skills are introduced through a retelling of the Myth of Psyche story, and caregivers tell their stories and describe difficulties in taking care of themselves.

Act Two focuses on selfcaring and selfhealing in the two major settings of our lives, our work and our home. We explore the work place, ways to work in a selfcaring way when relating to large scale organizations, and ways to have a selfcaring home life.

Act Three of the book deals with the practice and rehearsal of selfcaring, selfhealing skills in the four dimensions: physical, mental, emotional, and spiritual. We work with each dimension individually while recognizing in song and story that selfcaring and selfhealing require continuous integration of all four dimensions.

Act Four includes directions for designing your own selfcaring lifestyle and healing rituals. The appendix contains a sample ritual as well as Movements for Mending, references, and resource guides.

Throughout the book you will find poems, songs, and stories in contemporary language and conversational tone, along with, at times, a lighthearted spirit of humor. Not intended as irreverence to the importance of the topic, these are used to sustain us through what can be a hazardous dance. This book is called a "playbook" to suggest that work on your own selfcaring needs to be done in a playful spirit, and in brief segments of time. Give yourself permission after reading a section to put the book aside and let your inner creativity make connections to your life situations.

You will also find exercises and suggestions for steps to take on behalf of your own selfcaring and selfhealing. Some actions are a way of getting the most out of the book. Others can become an ongoing part of your daily life. In both cases, you will find your willingness to take action and use your kinesthetic senses to be the most powerful tool in creating your own learning.

Remember the Chinese proverb:

> *I hear, and I forget;*
> *I see, and I remember;*
> *I do, and I understand.*

Act One

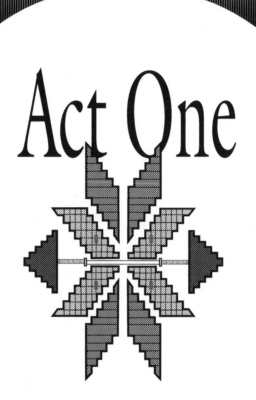

Steps, Techniques,
and Essential Elements

*In order to perform the dance of selfcaring/selfhealing, caregivers
must learn many steps and develop and practice many techniques.
Unfortunately, our early training (both personally and professionally)
only prepared us to do the movements of caregiving without regard for
ourselves. This means, in order to meet our needs as caregiving adults,
we are faced with the task of unlearning habits and techniques.*

*Most of our teachers and role models did not take care of themselves,
so they could not teach the dance of selfcaring. They may have spoken
of its value, but to become a dancer one must dance. To learn the
steps one observes and copies people who have the routine in their bodies, in
their bones. And mostly one needs permission to perform the ordinary
movements of everyday life in such a way that they won't interfere with
selfcaring, and result in setting up the need for selfhealing.*

*The first two chapters look at the change in our attitude towards taking
care of ourselves which is necessary to perform caregiving as
a healthy and graceful dance. We note the connection between the dance of
selfcaring and selfhealing and how, when you perform selfcaring
more often, you have less need for selfhealing. Caregivers tell their own stories
of how they often injured themselves as they performed their
caregiving work. We identify the essential selfcaring elements and offer
you, the reader, a way to identify which essential elements
may be missing in your life.*

The material for the dance is air,
the movement is breath,
and the source is love.

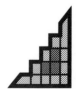

Becoming a Selfcaring, Selfhealing Person

1

Love thyself as thy neighbor.
Moshe Feldenkrais, *The Potent Self*

- Are you a person who takes care of others and has trouble asking for (or knowing) what you need for yourself?
- Do you treasure relationships, often putting up with people's lack of consideration for you?
- Do you often find, as you make and complete your "to do" list, that *your* needs are not even on your list?
- Do you dream of a world where all people will flourish?
- Do you feel uncomfortable (have trouble flourishing) when anyone you love is unhappy or in trouble?
- Are you a person who stays too long in a job or in a relationship out of a sense of loyalty, forgetting about the loyalty you owe to yourself?
- Do you go courageously to the front lines to tend the sick, wounded, and needy?
- Do you dream up projects to tend to the needs of the sick, wounded, and needy, and then get BLAMED as though you dreamed up the sick, wounded, and needy?

If you have answered "yes" to three or more of these questions, you are in need of learning the skills of selfcaring and selfhealing. In addition, you will probably need a lot of encouragement in putting selfcaring into your daily life. So find two or three friends and ask them these same questions. If they answer the same way you did, they are likely candidates to go on this journey of recovery with you. (We will go into more detail later on the importance of Partnership Power.)

In teaching professional helpers, I have encountered many people who would answer "yes" to most of the above questions. And even without asking, by scanning the facial expressions and body postures of the students before me, I can often guess how far they have strayed from selfcaring. Hunched shoulders, hyperextended necks, eyes straining to see as though through a thick fog, all testify to the effort and struggle that life has become.

Sometimes their selfcarelessness has amounted to a small miscalculation of limits and vulnerabilities or to an underestimation of what a particular project will require. Like the cafeteria diner with eyes bigger than stomach, we sometimes take on more than any human being could handle comfortably.

Susan, a nurse practitioner, had been experiencing headaches, tiredness, and a lack of her usual vigor. "Opening the new clinic was exciting, but it turned out to be all-consuming. Adding all the startup tasks on top of my regular work load has meant longer-than-ever work hours and a sense of going in all directions at once."

Other times selfcarelessness has gone on far longer, under more intense pressure. Robert, a former counselor put it this way: "I loved working with the clients in the beginning, but before it was over I wasn't doing them any good — or myself either. By the time I figured out what was happening to me, my burnout had cost me my marriage as well as my health."

So, selfcaring and selfhealing are intertwined. Impossible to separate at times, they dance back and forth as grapevines weaving around each other. As we desire to become more selfcaring, we discover the effects of prior injuries. As we attempt to heal, we notice our need to take better care of ourselves.

Selfcaring is a place halfway between selfless and selfish. Between the two extremes of the "saint" whose only regard is for others and the "sinner" who thinks only of himself, selfcaring is a place for regular people. Rather than taking a position of "them or me," selfcaring involves an inclusive sense of "and." Selfcaring means caring for oneself while, at the same time, caring for others.

Selfcaring Is Not:

- Continuing to educate and train ourselves to withstand more stress in order to take on more stress. We all know people who insist on staying in unhealthy jobs or relationships while asking for help in order to tolerate more abuse more gracefully.

- Putting ourselves through frequent recurring cycles of overwork, followed by crashing to recover. This rhythm of full speed ahead followed by total collapse is damaging to all dimensions of ourselves: the physical, mental, emotional, and spiritual.

Selfcaring Is Tuning In

...Recognizing, earlier and earlier, the subtle physical signs of potential difficulties.

- Caring people become good at reading other people's body language: clenched jaw, stooped shoulders, sad eyes. Selfcaring means tuning in to ourselves and learning how to read our own body language.

- Alcoholics don't have to wait to hit bottom on skid row before beginning their recovery. As we tune in earlier and earlier to ourselves and our own needs, we caregivers don't have to hit bottom— *we don't have to get sick in order to get well.*

Selfcaring Is Tending

- Being actively involved in a caring role creates the potential for taking on other people's tensions and stress. In tending to ourselves, we perfect the art of not taking on other people's tension. And when we do take on their tension, tending to ourselves we learn to let go quickly so we are free to experience a life of balance and vitality.

The selfcaring alternative, like all places of moderation and balance, is not easy to find, develop, and sustain over time. As we grow to become more selfcaring we discover our need to become selfhealing as well.

Selfhealing Is Not:

- Making unnecessary efforts from a desire to please, from the fear of making a mistake, or through the excess energy of our own enthusiasm. Our lives become graceful dances when we take out these extras and perform according to our own inner rhythm.

- Turning ourselves over to "experts." Whatever knowledge the specialists might have, I am the only *real* expert on me. You are the only expert on you. The self is not only the *object* of the healing but the *agent* of the healing as well. If we don't yet consider ourselves experts on ourselves, we can become so by applying the skills of selfcaring and selfhealing.

Selfhealing Is Making Whole

- Letting go of what is unnecessary while supplying the essential missing elements. When you were learning to write your name, it took great effort. It became easier when you learned to eliminate extra movements of your face and tongue and loosen your grip on the pencil. Eventually you made your signature legible.

- Unlearning the habits we acquired as we accommodated previous traumas. Recovery from a broken leg doesn't just involve getting the cast off. We must unlearn or let go of the way we have been walking to accommodate the cast.

- Transforming the pain in such a way that its truth becomes understandable. Pain is a signal that something is wrong, but the place where it hurts may not be the place where the difficulty lies. We can have pain in the shoulder or hips, the result of years of walking in poorly fitting shoes. Discovering the message in the pain involves listening to the wisdom of our bodies and taking steps to change the circumstances which have created the pain.

- Correcting imbalances whether in diet, body posture, work, or family. A lot of what we do to take care of ourselves really doesn't serve the purpose because we tend to overdo one or two favorite things. Selfcaring and selfhealing involve looking at the whole picture and discovering where omissions and excesses may be and moving towards balance.

The Kinesthetic Self

The connection between selfcaring and selfhealing finally occurred to me after many incidents of illness and recovery. I began to believe if I could take better care of myself in the first place, healing might not be needed so often.

And injury can come from the most unlikely places. After spending many years in the academic environment, I felt the need to heal after such intense emphasis on one particular way of thinking and experiencing myself and the world. It wasn't just that the logical, intellectual, and objective were emphasized. Most damaging to my spirit was the relentless ridicule of the intuitive. Subjective, felt experience was discounted and labeled "Touchy-Feelie."

In order to act on our own behalf we need to develop a sensitivity for reading the external messages in the environment. And we must be able to identify and name our own internal experience as well. Rather than running from the term "Touchy-Feelie," or regarding it as a vague insult, let's realize that these complementary parts of our kinesthetic senses are basic to our being, the stuff of which the dance is made. For the sake of precision and accuracy in our own selfcaring ability, let's exercise our power to name by using the word "Touchy" to represent our ability to make contact with the outer world, the world outside our skin. The term "Feelie" can be a name for our subjective inner experience, helping us connect with sensations and emotions. Instead of a vague label with negative connotations, "Touchy-Feelie" can be redefined as positive resources, to be respected and fine-tuned as we mature.

THE CREATIVE SELF

What if we had a culture that taught us, as children, to trust our sensory/motor system, our Touchy and Feelie senses? What if, as adults, we reclaimed our Touchy and Feelie senses and dared to trust our own experience? And how much better could we take care of ourselves if we knew how to communicate with our sensory/motor system? It is in this spirit, and to these ends, that I offer the following story.

As I was studying and writing about the kinesthetic senses, I remembered twin playmates I had as a child, unseen — but real to me. My parents called them "imaginary" and thought I invented them while Mother was preoccupied with my new baby brother. But perhaps this was my own creative way of connecting with Touchy and Feelie, of connecting with my own inner self.

I hadn't thought of my unseen playmates in years. But last summer, as I was studying and reading everything I could get my hands on about how our bodies, minds, and emotions function together, I thought of the twins again. As we became reacquainted, it was as though I were rediscovering parts of myself long hidden. Now let me introduce Feelie.

Feelie is highly sensitive and feminine, capable of a powerful inner focus which she uses, at times, to close off all other input and distractions. Her special skill is in noting small subtle movements within herself so that she is able to identify what she is experiencing. This is especially important in her own selfcare, in identifying her need for comfort and necessities such as food, water, and sleep. Feelie really knows who she is and where she is at any particular moment. Her special relationship to gravity keeps her well oriented in time and space.

If Feelie could speak for herself she would say, "I know up from down and all the other dimensions and directions by responding to my own inner signals. By sensing my internal organs and the experience of inner personal space, I recognize immediately when I'm off balance or when something I'm doing isn't good for me. I experience warmth, cold, pressure, and pain, and I'm especially fond of learning from pleasure."

When I remember Feelie from my childhood, I hear her full-bodied, heartfelt laughter. I love her sense of humor, her laughter at the slightest provocation. I'm reminded of Feelie whenever I hear the squeals and giggles of children.

Now let's meet Feelie's twin, Touchy. Touchy is strongly masculine and what you might call a mover and a shaker. He likes charging out into the world, contacting and sensing with his whole body. He learns about mountains by climbing, not by viewing them from afar.

Touchy is every bit as sensitive as Feelie. He notices pressure, heat, cold, and pain. He laughs a lot and may be even more fond of pleasure than Feelie. I admire Touchy's range and flexibility. He can move in every direction imaginable. In fact, if you look closely, you might notice the small, subtle movements of his muscles whenever he even *thinks* of moving in his mind's eye.

I see my friend Touchy as really knowing how to make contacts. He takes care of himself by moving out, using his own brand of detective skills to discover what's out there and what's needed to ebb and flow with it.

If Touchy could speak he'd say, "Most people don't realize that both Feelie and I process and organize a tremendous amount of information. Feelie is sensory; I am motor — and all stimulation of doing, learning, remembering, and healing are ordered by us, the sensory/motor systems."

As we learn to reconnect with our own twins (our sensory/motor systems), we learn we can trust them with our very lives. Let's call on the Soma Twins[1] for some background on how our misunderstandings about these senses have developed.

"Down through the ages we have been mistreated," said Touchy, "and the senses we represent relegated to a less important position than they deserve. Called evil, foolish, or the work of the devil at times, while at other times, we have been totally ignored. In western culture, we seem to get lost altogether for long periods of time."[2]

Feelie added, "The recent widespread practice of using drugs has been a source of concern, since people seem to think that is the way to get in touch with us."[3]

Responding to Feelie, I said, "One of the most misunderstood messages was a rallying cry for the faithful of the California cult: 'Experience ecstasy! Lose your mind and come to your senses!' Can you clarify this for us now?"

Both of the twins nodded at once, and Touchy said, "Stop leading with your logical mind. The logical part is designed to *follow* the body's sensing, feeling parts."

I was reminded of my ballroom dancing teacher, Eddie. He's always telling me, "Don't think, just follow!" And another dancing teacher gave this advice: "When spinning around, do not focus on the outer moving edges. Stay in the place in the center which is not moving. You'll be able to perform multiple turns at high speed without getting dizzy." This opens the possibility that you may contact your sensory/motor systems and, like the whirling dervishes, experience ecstasy without chemicals.

"At the very least," Touchy teased, "you will open up your sinus cavities, which is probably a prerequisite to experiencing ecstasy in any culture!"

On that note we leave Touchy and Feelie, my Soma Twins, knowing that we can call on them again to help us understand how they function, separately and together, to aid selfcaring and selfhealing.

THE FEMININE SELF

In all cultures and times, women have performed the dance of caregiving, feeding and caring for themselves in order to feed and care for their young. This dance, ancient and natural, has not been an easy one. Folk stories and myths have spelled out the difficulties of this continuing human dilemma — caring for oneself while staying in caring connection to others.

Steps in the dance of selfcaring are described in Greek mythology in the tale of Psyche. According to the story, in order for Psyche to be reunited with her husband from whom she had become separated, Psyche had to master several skills. She had to develop her own identity, learn how to get what she needs from an unfriendly world, ask for help for herself, and put limits on her helping of others. Psyche was given four tasks to complete. These tasks illustrate the five skills of selfcaring. These skills help to build and maintain strong boundaries between ourselves and those we care about.

THE FIVE SKILLS OF SELFCARING

1) SORTING AND SEPARATING what belongs to us from what belongs to others

2) LETTING GO AND SURRENDERING, and learning when and how to do this.

3) BUILDING and USING PARTNERSHIP POWER to get help from others

4) STEPPING BACK to see the big picture and the relationship between parts

5) EXERCISING CHOICE by SAYING NO and YES.

Let's retell the ancient Psyche tale with its archetypical view of the feminine helping role. We will look at each of Psyche's four tasks followed by the five selfcaring skills that are illustrated. In addition, we will examine a contemporary situation where each skill can be useful.

SELFCARING SKILLS AND THE MYTH OF PSYCHE

Meet Psyche, the pregnant mortal wife of the god Eros and daughter-in-law of none other than Aphrodite, goddess of love. As you can see from her illustrious relatives, this lady hung out in some mean company. Somehow she got separated from her husband just at the time she needed him the most, being pregnant and all. Since she was a mere mortal, she decided to throw herself on the mercy of her mother-in-law who was a goddess of pretty high rank and a known expert on this loving, caring business.

Why Aphrodite was out of sorts with her daughter-in-law isn't clear in the various versions of the story, and it isn't clear why she didn't just use her vast powers to set things right for the young couple. Instead, Aphrodite devised four extremely difficult tasks for Psyche to master before she could be reunited with her husband. As it turned out, these assignments were for Psyche's own good, teaching her the skills needed for selfcaring in personal, work, and family relationships. As you read about Psyche's struggles, ask yourself if you have developed these essential selfcaring skills in your own life.

TASK ONE: SORTING THE SEEDS

In her first task, Psyche was given a large pile of seeds of various types, all mixed together. She was told to separate them into piles according to whether they were oats or beans or barley seeds. Picture this poor woman, sitting at the table shuffling and grouping the seeds into separate piles, singing, "oats and beans and barley seeds, oats and beans and barley seeds." We can admire her grace in accepting such a meticulous and monotonous task.

Selfcaring Skill One: Doing Your Own Sorting Work

In reality, the tasks of sorting and separating our own seeds can be fascinating, fun, and enlightening. The seeds of our own discontent have been planted in our past, sowed by mother, father, grandparents, even by ancestors dead long before our birth. To sort out the messages of the past and to separate them from present people and realities means that we can choose which seeds we want to flourish in our own psyche. "One seed is from Mom, this one's from Dad. Don't forget Grandma. She always looked sad."

Contemporary Example: Your Own Sorting Work

Imagine yourself in the following situation. You are having a discussion with a friend, coworker or your boss. The outcome is important. The discussion and the person you are speaking with begin to stir old feelings, reminding you of someone else such as your ex-spouse, his bossy mother, or the boogie man! If you come on like gangbusters, reacting in this situation to feelings left over from another era, you are gonna get yourself in a whole lot of trouble. You will probably blow the deal, lose your friend, or hurt someone you love.

You need to sort out the seeds of the past and separate them from present reality. Imagine you can take two little wires, like brackets [ ], and place them around the memory, feeling, or issue that is emerging for you in the present context, and go on with the business at hand.[4] Make a note to deal with this later in a context that is appropriate for sorting the seeds of your own discontent. Keep in mind that unfinished business and unresolved situations drain energy. Ultimately doing your own psychological and emotional sorting work results in lightening your load. A caring lifestyle becomes easier as you no longer need to carry around the people and situations of the past.

Task Two: Gathering The Golden Fleece

The next task that Aphrodite presented to Psyche was to gather some golden fleece from a herd of mean, aggressive sheep. Now these were not those cute little fuzzy sheep that children cuddle or grownups count as they go off to sleep. We're talking about big bully rams, busy butting heads and locking horns with one another, over who knows what! Turns out, Psyche's no dumbbell. She doesn't even try to wrestle those rams or beat them at their own game. She waits until night when the rams have gone. Then she gathers the wool that stuck to the bushes where the rams were fighting and feuding with one another during the day!

SELFCARING SKILL TWO:
LETTING GO AND SURRENDERING

Many of us have given up our caring, helping, intuitive natures when confronted with head to head power plays. If you join the bully rams at their game, you lose your own way of being. There's also the risk of acquiring bruises and broken bones when playing war games. If you fight the power hungry rams or try to talk them out of their anger, you risk starting a stampede which will trample all gentle beings under hoof, including yourself.

CONTEMPORARY EXAMPLE:
LETTING GO AND SURRENDERING

Suppose you are sitting with a friend who is obstinate, complaining, and difficult. Whatever suggestions you make, they respond with, "yes, but..." You feel your energy draining from your body and imagine if you don't do something soon, you will need, at the very least, a complete energy transfusion. Rather than continuing these "going nowhere and using your own energy to *not* get there" movements, try de-escalating by LETTING GO (it's not going to happen your way, anyhow), SURRENDERING to whatever seems possible (go with the flow), and give up for now, as Psyche did so cleverly when she put things off until nightfall. ("You may be right, there may not be a solution to this situation.")

TASK THREE: FILLING THE FLASK

In order for Psyche to live a loving life with Eros, she had to fill a crystal flask with waters from a forbidden stream. The stream was guarded by dragons, and the whole thing looked hopeless until she asked an eagle for help. When Psyche was carried by the eagle, together they were able to back off from the scene and get a panoramic perspective. According to the ancient story, our heroine was then carried by the eagle to the stream, down past the dragons, where she filled the flask and they took off before they were discovered.

Selfcaring Skill Three:
Building and Using Partnership Power[5]

and

Self Caring Skill Four:
Stepping Back for a Broader Perspective

This task demonstrates two selfcaring skills. Instead of getting caught up with the barriers and becoming overwhelmed by the difficulty of a task, you may enlist the help of a friend. It's amazing how often those of us who help others forget to ask for help for ourselves. STEPPING BACK from a situation and getting a bird's eye view enables us to note patterns and significant details not obvious when viewed from close up. We can then move in quickly to accomplish what is necessary to sustain our own lives and to protect our significant relationships.

Contemporary Example:
Partnership Power And Stepping Back

So here you are, a gentle fair-minded soul, and some dingbat (parent, colleague, former friend, teenager) is abusing you. They are screaming, name-calling, and blaming you for all the ills of the last millennium. You find yourself shrinking inside. Part of you is picturing scenes of how you would like to see this person tortured and another part is believing what they are saying about you.

As you probably have noticed by now, not everyone operates from your value system of conscientiously helping and caring for others. Taking care of one's gentle soul in the presence of dragons calls for advanced selfcaring skills. This is especially true when you realize that, as in the myth of Psyche, dragons often guard the flowing waters of what is essential for our survival. In order not to take in the dragon energy and become like them or be run off by the fear of them, we must build strong, confident boundaries.

Selfcaring skills STEPPING BACK and PARTNERSHIP POWER can come to your aid. Backing off, imagine you are viewing the scene from a surveillance camera like the ones stores use to catch shoplifters. Get some assistance from your sense of humor by picturing the scene as a comic strip and the people, including yourself, as cartoon characters. Don't hesitate to call for assistance from passersby, friends or strangers, and your own Higher Power.

Task Four: Saying No To The Needy

The final and by far the most difficult task given Psyche by Aphrodite was to descend into the Underworld. Her assignment was to take a small box to the goddess Persephone and get her to fill it with some kind of beauty ointment. Now this doesn't sound too serious or difficult, but here comes the hard part. This gentle, loving woman is warned that she will be beseeched by pathetic people who will beg and plead for her help. Three times she must have the courage to stay on her own life's journey while people in need are pleading for her to stop and assist them. Should she allow herself to be drawn to help them, she will stay forever in the underworld and never become reunited with her husband.

SELFCARING SKILL FIVE: SAYING YES AND NO

In the musical "Oklahoma," when Ado Annie sang Rogers and Hammerstein's song "I'm Just A Girl Who Can't Say No," the audience was amused. But for a person who can't stay on his/her own life's path, the digressions are anything but funny. Saying "yes" and "no" must be a win-win situation both for ourselves and for the other person. From the perspective of selfcaring, we cannot say yes to another unless, in the same act, we are saying yes to ourselves.

CONTEMPORARY EXAMPLE: SAYING NO AND YES

Since setting limits and saying NO is such a difficult yet necessary skill, let's look at a number of situations where NO is the kindest answer you can give.

- A close friend wants you to: join his church, become president of the PTA, or run away with him to Nigeria. Your own life goals are in another direction so you say, "Thanks for the compliment, it was good of you to think of me." And "No, that isn't right for me."

- A relative, friend, or neighbor asks you for something and you give it to them. Instead of expressing gratitude he or she criticizes what you have done, and immediately thinks up something else for you to do to prove you really care. The only escape from this bottomless pit is to climb out quickly (surrender) and forgive yourself for falling into it in the first place. You say, "No, I'm sorry you haven't been pleased by my efforts and gifts. I've done all I can."

- Your son, spouse, or dearest friend is dedicated to living a reckless life of self-destruction by riding his/her motor-cycle without a helmet, drinking and driving, or continually ingesting illegal or over-the-counter-chemicals. As pitiful as this person seems, run, do not walk, to save your own life. Your response: "I'm history in your life. I will no longer hurt myself by watching you hurt yourself."

- A person has needed your care because of age, illness, or a situation of stressful overload. You have said yes to all his/her requests, and now it is time when, to rebuild confidence, the person needs to do for himself or herself. You respond, "No, I won't do it for you, but I'll support you in doing what you need to do for yourself."

You're probably saying to yourself, "If it were only as easy as it sounds!" To be in touch with one's own experience, to understand and define its meaning, and to act selfcaringly on one's own behalf takes discipline and **practice, practice, practice!**

*Dance is a delicate balance
between discipline and freedom.*

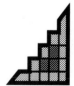

Caregivers and Their Caring Work

2

If caring is to be maintained, clearly the one caring must be maintained.
She must be strong, courageous and capable of joy.
Nell Nodding, *Caring*

"There is danger in the telling of the tale," I had been told, but I learned the meaning of this truth the hard way. I was directing my first workshop on selfcare for helping professionals. The participants were child welfare workers on society's front line. Their caring work involved investigating complaints of child abuse and neglect — when they weren't filling out paperwork or fighting with the cumbersome state system that employed them.

THE DANGERS IN CAREGIVING

We began the workshop logically, stating the problems of their caring work. I suggested to the participants: "Think about your work experience, a typical day or week, and about the situations that create for you the greatest difficulty. Perhaps it is a particular time of day when you seem to run out of steam or a situation which continues to repeat itself. 'Here we go again,' you may be saying to yourself. Imagine the type of situation where you feel the most vulnerable in your own selfcaring, a time when you wind up feeling drained, as though you have lost track of yourself."

"Paper work is what does me in!" said Donald. "I like the work, being with the clients, but the forms can drown you. The worst day is when I've set aside time to catch up, and an emergency comes along which has to take precedence. If I hadn't expected to do paperwork that day, it wouldn't have been so bad. But the fact of the matter is, there is no time to do the paperwork which is required of the job. I resent the feeling of this unfinished business hanging over my head and the dull headache I carry for days."

One of the women supervisors chimed in, "There are layers to this. As a supervisor I know the job is often impossible, but if the paperwork isn't done we lose workers. One unit didn't document all of their client contacts and they lost a worker because central office said they didn't need as many staff."

"I hate being the bad guy and having to say no to clients and staff when we don't have the resources," a Mexican American woman named Norma remarked. "Clients look up to you and expect that you can do anything, when in fact we are very limited."

"The hardest part for me is being the last resort," said Susan, a woman in her late twenties. "I'm the end of the line for the people who come to me. When kids have to be removed from their homes for their protection it's against the law to take them to the jail (the only local facility). The proper facilities are too far away from the rural community where I work. So late at night and on weekends, they drop them off at my home. This doesn't happen every weekend, but when it does, it means I have no time off from caretaking."

Dottie, a woman in her middle forties spoke up, "I used to do that but no more. I used to get so many calls at home, my husband put his foot down. Of course, since his mother came to live with us, I'm back to feeling I never have any time off anyway."

As group members continued complaining and commiserating with one another, sharing "war stories" and situations in which they felt most vulnerable, I felt a dramatic change in the energy in the room. Gone were the pleasant expectations of a day away from the office and the gentle curiosity about the workshop schedule. In their place was a dark discouragement bordering on despair. I imagined a sweat shop of the last century — workers chained to large machines, the cogs of great wheels grinding too slowly in spite of the workers' painful and costly efforts. This image of grinding prompted me to suggest a ten minute break for my own sake as well as for the sake of the participants. And then it hit me. In the telling of their tales, workshop participants were reexperiencing their work traumas and frustrations. They were reinfecting themselves and each other with feelings of hopelessness and helplessness about their work situations. No one in the room seemed to be breathing until I called time out.

When we reconvened I shared my "sweatshop fantasy" with the group and, amidst laughter and some nods of recognition, one woman seemed to be speaking for everyone when she made this comment: "It's like what they say about the weather, we all talk about it, but you can't do anything about it. When everybody sits around and bitches at my agency, this makes the problems worse for me. If I'm just left to do my job I'm fine, but it takes me two days to get over a staff meeting. We're called in and told about the pending budget cuts or the new policies, and it comes down to 'do more with less,' and we don't have any say about it anyway."

"How we are when we're together makes a tremendous difference for me in being able to take care of myself," Norma said. "I finally figured out that when I have lunch with a certain group of people, (I call them the 'doom and gloom boys'), I have no energy left for the afternoon."

At this point I suggested we all "circle up" (as in "circling the wagons") and join hands. I reminded each one to breathe and develop an inner focus while staying connected to the person on either side and, through them, to the whole group. I offered the following suggestions for selfcaring and selfhealing during our time together and in the future: "Appreciate yourself as a precious, valuable person who has chosen to do a difficult and sometimes impossible job. Because you can not do everything, take heart in doing what you *can* do for others and for yourself. Remember, you are not alone; others travel this caring path with you. Realize that the caring energy which has motivated you to be in these jobs can sustain you and help you to learn whatever is most needed for your selfcaring and selfhealing at this time in your life."

As the group members listened to my voice, they moved gently in rocking motions, nurturing themselves as one might soothe a distraught infant in the middle of the night. Our joined hands served to allow each person to experience connection with the larger group while staying centered in his/her individual rhythm. The rest of our time together went very differently from the beginning phase. The group meditation and affirmation that we did released us from living in and being overwhelmed by problems.

We began living in and experiencing solutions together. We began identifying the important missing elements in peopleworkers' lives. By the end of our time together the group members were sharing specific strategies they have used to include elements of selfcaring in their busy lives.

THE MISSING ELEMENTS

As I have continued to work with professional and non-professional helpers through the years I have heard many verses of what might be called "The caregivers' Lament." Not all peopleworkers have to deal with a large bureaucracy like the child welfare workers I've just described. Not all peopleworkers deal with life-threatening emergencies on a regular basis as they do. But in whatever setting or circumstances, we caregivers face our biggest challenge in finding ways to take care of ourselves.

In living a lifestyle where caring for others is central, essential elements such as *rest* and *recreation* can be missing. Or there can be an imbalance between two essential elements such as *work* and *play.* When one element is over-represented in our lives, something else vital to our selfcaring is being left out.

The child welfare workers, for example, were so caught up in the tremendous responsibility of their jobs and the serious problems in their work place that there was little sense of humor or true connection with one another. Sometimes there is too much *sound* and not enough *silence,* too much *abstinence* and not enough *nourishment.* And *movement* and *activity,* though vital elements, need to be balanced by opportunities for *stillness.*

One of the major themes of selfcaring is: it is possible to have too much of a good thing. Too much solitude may turn into isolation. Too much work means not enough play, resulting in a dull and joyless life in the short run. The long run effect can be burnout, sickness, and even death.

LAMENT OF THE CAREGIVERS

Let's listen to some other peopleworkers chanting their own unique verses of the caregiver's lament. Notice the common themes and how they reverberate with your own experience. As you read their stories, see if you can identify essential elements in the lives of the caregivers (such as work and play, sound and silence) which are out of balance or missing altogether.

"No wonder I'm a workaholic! My family and social life are in shambles!"

Cynthia is a 43 year old marriage and family therapist. She has a large, successful practice and supervises and trains other professionals. "I finally got the divorce I should have gotten years ago, and I'm OK about that. It took a lot for me to admit I couldn't save my own marriage when I have been so successful in helping other people to save theirs. But I got past that. The problem now seems to be, how do I develop a whole new personal and social life when I am so involved in my work? I feel I need permission to take time out for myself without getting sick to do it."

Cynthia touches on several themes familiar to many helping professionals. We know, for balance in our lives, a well rounded social and personal life is critical. But it's often not as easy as it sounds. When the element of *work* is not balanced with *play,* less effective work results and finally illness. Being sick is one way to get a guilt-free day off, but it's a lousy way to have to spend it.

Relationship difficulties in our personal and family lives are particularly challenging for those of us whose work involves helping others. Our need to work things out with spouses, children, and friends can go far beyond other people's willingness to invest in that process. And some difficulties occur precisely because of our professional work. When my daughter was an adolescent she found a clever way to discount me. Whenever I was trying to negotiate with her regarding some difficulty we were having she would say, "I don't want any of that '*social work*' talk." When the son of a minister friend of mine got As in all school subjects except religion, which he flunked, I started to catch on.

"*If I don't stop taking responsibility for everyone, I'm going to burn up!*"

Ralph is an ambitious, successful psychologist in his middle thirties. As part of his vacation plans he had elected to participate in a workshop on selfcare for helping professionals. "It's hard to give up what I'm good at. I'm a good listener. In fact, people pay me a lot of money to listen to them. My heart feels open to people, and I like that, but I take it in my gut. I feel so much responsibility, it can be overwhelming. Before I left town last Friday, I was running around like crazy trying to see everybody and get my clients all taken care of so I could have a week's vacation. Now I have to recover first before I have the energy to enjoy my time off."

Ralph's variation of burnout he describes as "burning up." A moth is attracted to the flame but it doesn't have the intelligence to stop at a safe distance. Becoming selfcaring means developing the ability to stop and to pace ourselves so we do not continue cycles of overdoing followed by time out for healing and recovery. Selfcaring means noticing earlier and earlier how we are using ourselves so we can interrupt the patterns before we do irreversible damage to ourselves. The openness of Ralph's heart serves him well as a helping person, but he needs the skills to be empathic to his *own* needs and to listen to himself as well as to others. The important element of *rest* may need to come before *recreation*, and these, like the other elements, need to be in balance with one another before selfcaring and selfhealing can occur.

"The work gets so heavy, continually dealing with issues of life and death"

Ann is a registered nurse who had worked five years in the oncology ward with children who had cancer. "I found that work very rewarding but I had to give it up a year ago. I'm working in the labor and delivery room now where we have more good news than bad. I still have trouble with the bad things that happen to good people. Often I can't get patients off my mind after the shift is over. In addition to that, we have to deal with the politics of the hospital. When I see what little budget support we get from the administrators and all the political infighting among groups, I just want to run away and join the circus."

One of the gifts we receive in witnessing birthing and dying is a clear understanding of what really matters. Recognizing what matters can establish, personally, a balance between the elements of *seriousness* and *humor*. Since many work organizations are not operating from a place of balanced perspective, maintaining our own balance can be even more difficult. Like Ann, many of us see clearly what is wrong in our work place and may have ideas to correct the situation. Recognizing that the work world isn't the way we want it to be — and it's not about to shape up to our liking any time soon — we can decide what to take seriously and act upon and when to laugh and enjoy the ludicrous nature of the situation. (*humor*) And regretfully, there are situations which require leaving one's worksite or even one's occupation for the greater interest of selfcaring and selfhealing. (*letting go*)

"When the client expresses emotion and cries, I lose touch!"

Daniel is a massage therapist. He says, "I enjoy working with people, relieving their stresses and strains. I love to see the difference in people as they come in, tired and worn out, and as they leave, relaxed yet energized. However when the client cries, I have trouble. I've always felt uncomfortable around someone crying. It probably goes back to the time after my Dad left. My mother used to sit in her room and sob for hours. I felt so helpless. Now, when a client starts to cry, I find myself wanting to end the session as quickly as I possibly can."

Daniel is pointing out some of the key rewards and costs of being a professional helper. We often have the privilege of witnessing people's growth and transformations. And, as part of this process, we witness their fears and pain. *Pleasure* and *pain* are both essential elements for selfcaring and selfhealing.

As Daniel described it, when someone else's expression of emotions hooks into our own unresolved pain from the past, we're confronted with our own "demons." Intense work with people demands a willingness to face our own issues from the past.

The choices are to see this as an opportunity to grow and learn or to run for safety to another profession, one that doesn't involve such intense people contact. But not being one who earns a living as a helper doesn't mean that we are free from the strains of helping roles. Most of us spend a great deal of time caring for relatives. Meet Lisa.

"I'm just the cook, maid, chauffeur, and laundry woman!"

Lisa is an attractive mother of three children ages 10, 12, and 16. She is a full time mom, a volunteer for her church, the wife of a professional man , and the only daughter to a father whose health is poor. "I've always wanted to be a mother, and I do think it is an important job. And I want to do right by my Dad at this difficult time in his life. But there sure are times when I don't think anybody sees me except for what I can do for them. I give, give, give and they take, take, take. I want something for myself, something that doesn't involve being somebody's relative. And I long for some time to myself with no one wanting anything from me."

For most of us, our connections to others provide significant enrichment to our lives. But for our own selfcaring and selfhealing, these *connections* must be balanced by *solitude*, by quiet time to listen and respond to our own inner needs.

Healthy giving needs to be balanced by receiving. If not, our giving actions create resentment towards the very people who mean the most to us. In longing for a time when nobody will want anything from her, Lisa personifies the problem we codependent caregivers have in giving *ourselves* permission for our own selfcaring. As long as we are connected to many others, we'll never run out of relatives, nor will the relatives run out of wants for us to fulfill.

Selfcaring and selfhealing require that we demand time for ourselves (*solitude*) regardless of whether people need things from us or not. Training others to take over and relieve us from our family duties may be one of the most important steps in making selfcaring possible and in reducing our need for selfhealing. (*support* and *connection*)

"They just won't take responsibility for their own health!"

Gary, a participant in a selfcare workshop began describing his biggest problem as a dentist. "The hardest situation for me is when patients don't take their dental health seriously. They wait till they get a toothache in the middle of the night, and then expect me to fix the damage. Even when I explain it to them, some will listen and some will continue to expect me to fix them up after the damage is done. Recently I've made the connection between the backaches I get at the end of the day and the patients I see. When I see those frustrating patients, I go home with a backache. Other days I can work long hours with no trouble. Another thing I know about myself that seems related here —I want my patients to like me, and I'm sure that is part of the problem."

In the health care field, practitioners talk about "patient compliance." People are considered "good" patients and clients when they do what the doctor says. We are making trouble for ourselves when we expect our students, patients, (or children for that matter), to do what we say because we say it. The missing element here seems to be a balance between *support* and *challenge* in the partnership between helper and helpee. Gary supports his patients in taking care of their teeth and accepts the challenge of getting his message across. But having done his part, Gary needs to pass the challenge of caring and healing on to his patients who are the only ones who have the power to accomplish it.

Gary's backaches suggest that he needs to *support* himself in not taking on that which he can't do anything about. Becoming more selfcaring may require *challenging* himself to set limits on his helping habits. Selfcaring for helpers sometimes requires withdrawing our services, without malice, from people who have demonstrated an inability to benefit from our help.

"I feel I need some 'soul healing' myself."

Ted had been a psychiatrist for 20 years and will be 50 next month. Ted explained, "The word psychiatry comes from a Greek word that means 'soul healing,' and that's what I'd like to order for myself. Maybe the problem is my age or too many years with too many people who are too sick to heal. Whatever it is, I feel stuck. Managing two offices and running back and forth between two hospitals feels like too much. Getting a car phone has made it easier to keep up with my phone calls, but now there's no quiet time. Even the patients seem all alike at this point, and I find myself wondering, is this why I went into medicine?"

It is possible to have too much of any good thing, and Ted's comments illustrate several elements of selfcare out of balance in this way. He is sensing his age has something to do with his discontent , and that seems quite likely. We can expect the proper balance between *movement* and *stillness,* or *variety* and *routine*, or *challenge* and *support* to be different at different times in our lives. What may have been exciting and challenging in Ted's 30's and 40's now may seem dull and routine.

Technology and specialization have created some problems for caregivers while it solved others. Like freeze-dried soup, it's efficient, but it's not as delicious or nutritious as the old-fashioned kind. The element of variety is missing when professionals and agencies specialize in serving one type of client or one problem condition. Burnout takes place faster when there isn't enough variety in the ways we use ourselves or in the types of challenges we are confronting. On the other hand, little comfort is received from routines which allow no time for human contact and support from coworkers and staff.

"I always went to workshops to learn things for my clients. This time I'm here for me."

Nancy is a psychiatric nurse who specializes in working with chemically dependent patients and their families. "I want to know how to stay emotionally in touch with the patients without becoming drained myself. Let's face it. Some of the people I work with are not pleasant to be around, especially in the early stages of their recovery. I find myself withdrawing behind my paperwork, but then even my staff feels shut out. I receive a lot from contact with some of the patients, but I guess I don't know how to keep clear boundaries without erecting a wall."

Bringing the focus back to herself is an important step in Nancy's selfcaring. She is recognizing that the workshops are not only for what she can learn to help her patients, but for her own benefit. Our needs count too, and, in the long run, taking care of ourselves means we are better able to carry out our caring work.

Keeping clear boundaries between ourselves and others without erecting a wall involves finding a balance between *taking in* and *letting go*, knowing what we need for our own *nourishment* in relationships, and withdrawing when it is time for *abstinence*.

"Both my husband and I are workaholics!"

"We've teased about it for years, but it's nothing to joke about," Maureen, a social worker in her late forties told me. Maureen's voice was shaky, and tears rolled from the corners of her eyes as she made this admission to herself and to me. "The other morning I woke up angry at my husband, Jeff, who runs his own insurance agency. After we both had promised to stop over-working, he was leaving the house early for the third day in a row on top of having gotten home late the night before. We keep taking on more and more until we have no time together, no time for ourselves, and no energy left for enjoyment when we do get a day off."

Maureen continued, "Jeff and I did have a good talk over the phone after our angry words this morning. We both realized that we have the habit of just 'trying harder' when things start happening at work. Jeff gets anxious about money if he's not working overtime, and I start overdoing when I think people's needs aren't being met. We both seem to believe that if each of us does everything right, nothing will ever go wrong at work. Like other addictions, controlling our workaholism seems impossible. Jeff told me he kept saying the Serenity Prayer to himself after our argument: 'God, grant me the serenity to accept the things I cannot change, courage to change the things I can, and the wisdom to know the difference'." [1]

The problem with having work as an addiction is that it *appears* so worthwhile. We are filling a need, accomplishing something, and earning money in the process. But eventually, when we've done too much of this good thing, we hurt ourselves and those around us. There's no time or energy for *play* or *rest* or *relaxation*.

Maureen and Jeff have come a long way already in seeing their difficulties as a kind of addiction. Like people who realize that their drinking has gotten out of hand, they vow to control it. They make a plan, but gradually their resolve slips, and before long the drinking (or overworking) is back where it was before.

In order to become selfcaring, we peopleworkers, like Maureen and Jeff, must learn to set realistic boundaries on our working habits and stick to them. Like people who overdo with drugs or alcohol, those of us who overdo in our work can benefit from a twelve-step program to deal with our workaholism and our addiction to helping others.

YOUR CONTINUUM OF SELFCARING ELEMENTS

How balanced are some of the key selfcaring elements in your life? A balanced life, like a balanced diet, means that we don't have too much of any one thing while experiencing a deficiency of other necessary elements. Selfcaring and selfhealing result when we discover what we need and find ways to include it in our lives, keeping in mind the need for balance.

People who have a problem maintaining optimum weight often use food to satisfy other (non-nutritional) needs. Food can be used for comfort, to energize, or to reward yourself. Food can also be a way to avoid experiencing and dealing with unpleasant feelings. Stuffing ourselves with food can be a way of stuffing our feelings as well.

We can overdo other things besides food. Often we have too much of a good thing as we tend to rely on one activity, substance, or relationship to fill all our needs. Maybe it's jogging or aerobics or gambling or sex or alcohol or other drugs. We can overdo work using work or helping others in our personal life to give us a sense of worth, security, and identity. The list of potentially addictive things is endless, but the damaging result to our selfcaring and selfhealing is the same.

We can interrupt this pattern of using something as our one and only "fix" by identifying what element is missing. Rather than thinking of a "fix," like an on-off light switch, imagine a continuum (like a rheostat) between related selfcaring elements. Rather than thinking of good elements which we continually want to increase in our lives and bad elements which we work to avoid — think of all of life's elements as necessary, each with its own benefit, each with its own part in our balance. When we don't feel own own pain, we cannot identify when something is wrong. When we feel only pain we miss out on life's pleasures. Time alone can be important to our selfcaring, but too much turns into isolation. Experiencing connection to others is one of the things that life is about, but when we don't have time to ourselves, we have less and less to give to others. Use the following self-test to see where you are at this point in time in relation to some key selfcaring elements.

● ●

Selfcaring Elements: A Self-Test

On each of the following lines, place an **X** to represent where you are today in regard to each of the pairs of elements listed. If the two elements on the same line feel in balance right now your **X** will be near the center. If one of the elements is overrepresented in your life at the present time, your **X** will be closer to that element and further away from the one which is underrepresented.

movement ....stillness
work ....play
nourishment ....abstinence
seriousness ....humor
pleasure ....pain
challenge ....support
solitude ....connection
variety ....routine
recreation ....rest
taking in ....letting go

Notice the elements which seem most absent from your life. In the space below identify ways to include them, avoiding ways which are immoral, illegal, or fattening.

_____

_____

_____

Go back and circle the element(s) that you want to focus on especially for the coming week. Remember, balance and harmony are your goals, so take care not to take on too many elements at one time. Next week you can take the self-test again and see what a difference the missing element(s) has made in the balance of your continuum of selfcaring. Since this is not an exhaustive list you may want to add your own elements as you become more familiar with this way of thinking.

Remember, each time you complete the test you have created a snapshot of one point in time. To get a moving picture of your patterns over time you will need to repeat the test on a regular basis for a while and compare your results.

BE AWARE OF REMEDIES

We started this chapter with the caution that there is danger in the telling of the tale. Let's finish by remembering there is danger in *remedies* as well as in the ways they are administered. The above instrument and any of the other tools and techniques suggested in this book are just that. Use them as suggestions. Allow them to stimulate your thinking in a different direction or to interrupt your usual pattern of behaving. Use them gently, with kindness to yourself. If you find something here which doesn't move you in the direction of selfcaring and self-healing, or if and when it outlives its usefulness, discard it and create your own. You are the only *real* expert on you and your own experience — your most reliable guide.

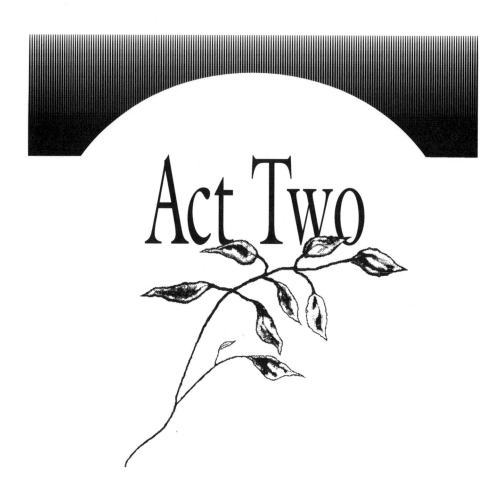

Act Two

Stage
and Settings

*T*he caregivers' dance of selfcaring/selfhealing cannot be a solo,
limited to private spaces and times we are alone. Caregivers perform a communal
dance, in step with others in the work place and at home. Attending to the
setting where caregiving happens helps us identify whether we have the necessary props
to perform our roles. We ask, does the place where we do our work support us
as well as supporting what we are trying to accomplish there? For caregivers whose work
place is also their home — is there a place for privacy, wings behind which
you can be offstage? And what of the supporting cast? The intricate dance of
balancing our own needs with the needs of others may receive little
applause unless we carefully select partners, friends, and colleagues who know
how to take care of themselves.

In the next three chapters we look at the subtle (and not so subtle) aspects of the
stage and setting where we perform the movements of our daily lives.
We look at actions to take and situations to avoid so we may move gracefully
and harmoniously in our offices and homes, and (for some of us) in our
relationship to large organizations.

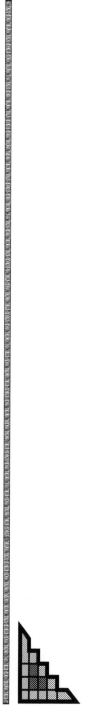

*Dance is the only art wherein
we ourselves are the stuff
of which it is made.*

A Selfcaring Work Place

3

Mary, Mary, quite contrary, how does your garden grow?
With silver bells and cockle shells, and pretty maids all in a row.
                    Mother Goose nursery rhyme

The question that no one has bothered to ask here is, why is Mary so contrary? Is she not happy with the silver bells of her telephone, her typewriter, her copy machine, her data processing screen? How about the door bells she answers to welcome the cockle shells, and the maids a-typing in their rows. Perhaps rocks and weeds are crowding out her seedlings, and neighborhood roughnecks have been digging up her bulbs and trampling her blooms. Unlike the nursery rhyme, it must be here stated that having telephones to ring and little maids (and men) to answer them does not a working garden make.

We are on the right track if we think of spaces and places where we work as gardens. People, like plants, can only bloom where they are planted if conditions exist to support growth. In this chapter we will be looking at the important conditions necessary to do the dance of selfcaring, selfhealing in the work place. First we explore the match between the person you are and the type of work you are doing. Next we look at the physical environment and how the work space itself contributes to or detracts from the type of work you are attempting to accomplish there. We look at low budget efforts you can make to help your work place become more compatible with your needs. Finally, we discuss some actions to enable you to work in a selfcaring way.

THE CRITICAL MATCH

Just because we are able to do certain work doesn't mean it is the right work for us. The importance of the match between a person and the type of work he or she does was taught to me by a client I will call Matthew.

MATTHEW'S DISCONTENT

When Matthew was 35 years old he came to me expressing extreme dissatisfaction with his work life. He performed his job well, giving each task caring attention. His supervisors and employers were pleased with his performance. His family told him that he'd better hold on to his good job since good jobs are hard to find these days. But still he felt unfulfilled and unhappy.

While he was in a state of deep relaxation, I asked Matthew to go back and remember what ideas he had about work when he was a little boy. He remembered playing with trucks and blocks and erector sets and, in the voice of his younger self, he said, "Work means to build things that last."

And why was Matthew's present job such a mismatch with who he really is? Each day he stocked merchandise on shelves from which people on the next shift filled orders. Each day when he returned to work, his finely organized patterns, the symmetrical rows he had carefully constructed, were all destroyed. No mystery his discontent, this assault to his soul each day of his work life.

Ideally, *you* have a better match between your values about work and the actual work that you do. If you don't, and the mismatch is anywhere near as troubling as Matthew's, the most selfcaring, selfhealing act you can perform is a career change. Caring peoplework can be rewarding and fulfilling, but not if you have always wanted to be a forest ranger or a deep sea diver.

If we continue with the analogy of the work place as a garden and people as the plants that try to bloom there— consider yourself, through the magic of your own imagination, in a waltz of the flowers.

• •

WALTZ OF THE FLOWERS: A FLOWER FANTASY

What if you were a valuable, delicate plant in need of a specific type of environment to enable you to survive and thrive? Do you know what type of plant you are and what conditions are necessary for your own blooming? Read through the following exercise, and then give yourself the gift of a few minutes to explore the activity on your own.

Consider the incredible variety of types of flowering plants! There are tall and short shrubs and shy and bold flowers. You will find brilliantly colored blooms growing in likely and unlikely places, singly and in clusters, on broad meadows and narrow ledges.

When you walk through a garden, notice not only the variety of flowers but the variety of their preferred surroundings as well. There are sunny and shady spots and a variety of soils, dry and sandy or moist and mossy. While some types of flowers thrive best in rock gardens, others need marsh lands or a small pond for their best nourishment. While some plants need frequent watering, others, like the cactus, store their own water from one season to the next.

Some flowers bloom all summer, others in fall, others bloom only once every few years. And plants have many ways of relating to the environment as well. Some vines need latticework to climb. Others, like Texas bluebonnets, send chemicals into the soil to change the surrounding area. This causes other plants to die back and give the bluebonnets needed room.

Even amateur gardeners can tell you that whatever knowledge you have of soils and fertilizers, of sprinkling systems and weather conditions, the major mystery in creating a successful garden is the locating of particular plants in the place where their needs are met.

So imagine yourself as a flower.
- Do you notice a sturdy stalk or stem, or do you see yourself climbing a wall or an arching cornice?
- Do you thrive in the summer heat, or do you fare better in sheltering shade?
- Are you able to bloom in a window box overlooking a city street? Perhaps you would feel more at home in a terracotta container on the back patio.
- Do you do better surrounded by other flowers, or are you a loner bud who likes lots of elbow room?
- How about being planted in rows and neat, straight lined beds — or would a random pattern suit your temperament best?
- What type of head gardener or nursery person would you like? Someone who plots and plans down to the smallest detail or one who tills and sows, provides plenty of fertilizer and then lets nature take its course.

Allow images of flowers and gardens, pictures of parks and nature settings to appear in the window of your inner mind. Appreciate and enjoy the images of the various types of flowers until you notice that one particular image keeps returning to you. After you have discovered your attraction to this special species of flower, imagine yourself as that flower. Describe yourself as that flower.

"I am a (name flower).
My petals are _____.
I grow best in _____ and with _____.
I need lots of _____ and I especially
enjoy_____."

Take note of what you have discovered about yourself in this flower fantasy. This image of yourself as a flower comes from the right side of your brain and may contain information that is not available when using only the left, or analytical side.

Share what you experienced in this fantasy with someone who knows you well. It also might be fun to look up the official description of the flower you visualized in your fantasy. What does it require to grow and bloom? What steps do you need to take in your work life to insure that you can blossom and enjoy the successful outcome of your labors?

YOUR OWN WORK PLACE

When you feel certain about the kind of flower (worker) you are, and you have a match between yourself and the type of work you are doing, it's time to think about the *place* where you do most of your work. What does this place feel like, this place where you spend so much of your time? Is it nourishing — or draining of your energies?

Do you ever see the light of day, the natural light so necessary for plants and other living things? How far do you have to go for a breath of fresh air? What is the view from your work station? Restful? Boring? Invigorating?

What about sound? Noise pollution can be draining as you work to screen out distracting sounds. On the other hand, the sound of falling water or some "white noise" machines can invoke a restful meditative state that aids concentration.

Listen as a group of peopleworkers discuss with me their work-places, the places where caring, helping, and healing is supposed to happen.

After the group had taken a few minutes to image themselves as flowers and then to picture their current work environments, Judith began the discussion.

"I pictured myself as a water lily in a quiet, cool, shady pond. When I think about my work environment, I see the color orange. That's the color they have painted the staff areas of the hospital where I work. The activity in these areas is hurried and hectic, and, of course, very crowded. In the areas where the patients are, care has been taken to have relaxing colors, but in the *trenches*...!"

"It's the same thing at the facilities where I consult," Chris remarked. "Sometimes I ask myself, if I'm suppose to have so much authority, how come I don't have a place to sit down?"

Helen added her discoveries from the exercise. "I realize just how bad some of my working conditions are. In the adult day care centers where I work, the buildings are old, and the heating and cooling is difficult to regulate. In the summer, the temperature is often over 90 degrees, and I am trying to do activities with twenty-one people in not nearly enough space."

"The temperature in new business buildings isn't that easy to regulate, either," I said. "I was presenting a seminar for bank employees in the late afternoon, after the bank had closed to the public. As I was speaking to the staff in the main lobby, the area was becoming hotter and more uncomfortable by the minute. When I inquired, I was told that the air conditioning was on a timer controlled from downtown. So, when the customers leave, the Texas heat is allowed to enter."

"Sends quite a message of management's regard for their employees," Mark, a rehab counselor said.

"I was thinking of the air in the building where I work," Susan remarked. "It's better now that they don't let people smoke at their desks, but the air still gets stuffy and stale. And of course, when they remodeled our building they fixed the windows so you can't open them."

"When you mentioned not having a place to sit down to review records, I thought about the nightmarish furniture in the places where teaching and learning is supposed to be taking place," a high school teacher, Dennis, said. "It seems like I'm forever moving furniture, unless, of course, I get one of those classrooms where the chairs are bolted to the floor!"

"When I imagine my ideal work environment, I see plants and sunlight and hear natural sounds of water and birds," Shirley said. "In contrast, in the real world, I have on several occasions had offices without windows."

"In one counseling center where I worked in an office without windows, I took some pretty drastic action," I told the group. "I turned my desk to the corner, and, in the open triangle between the walls and my desk, I brought in a bunch of plants. I rigged grow lights from the ceiling to keep the plants alive, and, as the plants flourished, it did wonders for my spirit."

THE POWER OF THE PHYSICAL ENVIRONMENT

Visiting with Ralph Caplan, a designer writer who consults on work spaces, I came to appreciate the power of the environment to affect our comfort level, our ability to focus and concentrate, and, finally, our sense of ourselves. Caplan has said it well in some poems he wrote for an ad campaign to promote office systems.

Everybody needs a Here.
A nest, a niche,
a room of one's own.
A space with enough
of its own character
to accept yours.
A corner that belongs to you
as much as you belong to it.

Somewhere you know
that knows you:
a homeroom at school,
a familiar street, a ship in port.

Anywhere that welcomes
you back when
there is no one there to say it.
A sense of place, solid enough
for light to break against.

No one wants to be nowhere.
Or closed in.
Any environment is wrong
if you feel stuck in it.
A sense of place,
a sense of light
and openness,
a sense of choice.
These are qualities we seek
in the spaces where we live.
And work.[1]

"Nobody smokes in church," Ralph reminded me," and people don't find it necessary to put up 'no smoking' signs, either! The design of a church communicates to people the kind of behavior that is expected there. In the work place the environment encourages certain types of behaviors, such as collaboration or discussion or solitary concentration. Or the environment discourages such activities."[2]

The physical spaces of a work environment may drain us or be supportive of our energies, depending on the match between the kinds of situations encouraged and the type of work we are attempting to perform there. If your work calls for private, confidential conversations, partial walls open to the ceiling will seem a threat. A space with no windows or outside light source, while providing privacy, could easily seem like a prison cell.

A Selfcaring Workplace

"With all the studies on color and its effect on mood, the most important factor may be whether people can pick the color, whether people have even the illusion of choice," Ralph continued in our discussion on creating healthy work environments.

"Since the environment has such a strong impact on us, even dictating our behavior at times, to be selfcaring we need to consider the environment and make what choices we can about it," I said.

"Yes, probably one of the worst things that can happen in life is to feel stuck, and in the work place people often don't exercise the potential choices which are there," Mr. Caplan concluded.

Taking care of one's self in the work place sometimes means acting on your own behalf to change or alter your working environment. Like the plants that send chemicals into the soil to create a better place for their own growing, you may need to alter aspects of your physical work environment. EXERCISING CHOICE is a selfcaring skill as well as a significant part of work satisfaction.

Look at the physical environment around you and discover what changes need to be made in order that your work space fits you and the work you do in it. As an example, let's start with something basic. What about the chair you are sitting in?

What's In A Chair?

Most people are conscious of the need for a good night's sleep and of the important role a good mattress plays in meeting this need. But what about the work chairs that we sit in, often for extended periods of time, day after day, year after year? Whether working at a desk or driving a car, our sense of place and our experience of support depends on some type of chair.

Lower back pain is the most frequent cause of absenteeism in the work place, and the chairs we sit in are major contributors to this ailment. Yet people often object to spending a bit more money for chairs which have been designed with the human frame in mind.

Sitting in most chairs means that we give up our own self support. By sitting in chairs with the so-called "bucket" design, we collapse into cushions which feel comfortable initially. But like the too-soft mattress, we don't get enough support and we are exhausted at the end of the day. After months and years of living like this, we lose the ability to support ourselves in a sitting position. What is needed in a chair is a supportive structure which encourages supporting oneself.

Chairs, like people, come in all sorts of shapes and sizes. Unfortunately, the shapes and sizes of chairs do not always correspond to the shapes and sizes of people. Like shoes, there is no substitute for trying the chairs on, moving around in them and pulling them up to a workstation. Remember too, no chair is good for your body for very long, so plan to take breaks and change positions often. For some questions to ask as you select your own supportive chair see Appendix A, Guide For Selecting A Chair.

MORE ABOUT YOUR PHYSICAL ENVIRONMENT

After you have secured a flexible yet supportive chair, the next consideration is your work station. Here, too, flexibility is important in your ability to take care of yourself. Where is your telephone located? Do you have to strain to reach it? Is your position awkward as you hold the phone to your ear? In balancing the elements of movement and stillness, it helps if the furniture and equipment can be adjusted to suit your size and the body positions which are comfortable for you.

Speaking of the telephone, peopleworkers often spend lots of time with the phone. It's in one hand or the other or tucked under the chin. It's not only those actual conversations but those many hours of playing telephone tag, returning calls from people who are returning your calls, etc. which add up to total telephone time. Try the following exercise, created by Ilana Rubenfeld, to increase your awareness of how you relate physically with your telephone.

SELFCARE AND THE TELEPHONE*

Imagine you hear the phone ring but don't answer at once. Notice how you feel. Do you hold your breath? Are you getting ready as if expecting the worst? As you reach for the phone do you stick your head and neck out? Do you always hold the phone with the same hand and crunch it against your shoulder? Are you tired after you put the phone down? Stop and notice next time you are actually answering your phone. You can't change habitual patterns unless you're aware of what you're doing. Here are some guidelines for selfcare while using the phone.

1. When you hear the first ring, take a deep breath and don't answer.
2. Place both feet on the floor so you will be balanced.
3. Don't reach for the phone with your head and neck. Stop first, then reach with your hand, leaving your body sitting back in the chair and keeping your head and neck loose.
4. Take the receiver and bring it to your ear without tilting your head. Keep your head balanced and in the middle.
5. After a few minutes, change hands and put the receiver to the other ear.

* (Exercise from Ilana Rubenfeld in *Women and Work, 1985*) [3]

If your work involves *extensive* time on the phone consider investing in (or requesting that your company provide) a telephone headset. It frees both hands for your work and relieves the stress which can build up in neck, shoulder, arm, and hand muscles.

What About Lighting?

Now that you can be comfortable on the phone, what about lighting? When I interviewed designers of work spaces, they named light as the first and most important consideration for healthy worksites. I asked the question, "If you didn't have much money to spend, what suggestions would you make to improve a work environment?" The answer came back, "Focus on your lighting! Replace florescent lights with full spectrum bulbs (lights which contain all the colors of natural sunlight) and use task lighting." (Task lighting spotlights the area where light is needed for particular tasks.)[4]

Many of us remember, when we were children, teachers and parents reminding us of the importance of having enough light on our books and papers. Insufficient lighting creates eye strain which causes headaches which take a lot of the fun and pleasure from our work day.

With the advent of computer screens, flexibility in light sources has become an important matter also. A small change in the angle of light hitting the screen or paper in front of us can conserve the energy we might be wasting staring and straining to see.

A MORE COMFORTABLE WORKPLACE

Speaking of seeing, what is your view from your work station? We want protection from distractions, but a lack of visual stimulation in the environment is not the answer either. And what about sound? Let's ask some other peopleworkers to discuss what they have done to give their work spaces a sense of place, to create a feeling for themselves of being "at home" where they work!

Sharon, a manager for a retail company began telling the group of her experiences in the corporate world. "Some companies and work organizations won't allow employees to decorate their offices with personal items because it takes away from the corporate image they are trying to portray. I can appreciate the need for some consistency in the overall design of the building, but it's important for me that my office reflect something of who I am and what I do there. I always bring a few items from home to give me a sense of continuity and the comfort of familiar surroundings."

"I like being able to surround myself with pictures that have some personal meaning to me," Susan, a drug abuse counselor commented. I like pictures of my family, along with some pictures that remind me of places where I have felt especially good, like the mountains or the sea shore."

"I have a sandbox in my office," the psychologist Ralph boasted. "Well, 'box' is a bit of an exaggeration. It's actually an old ash tray that, when we went to a smoke-free work place, I filled with sand and miniature stones and shells from my trips to the beach. Not only does it remind me of a favorite spot, but I can recapture some of that mellow 'beach feeling' playing with the sand between my fingers while I'm returning phone calls."

"Music is an important way for me to stay in a mellow place," a nurse, Ruth Ann admitted. I always found it helpful to play tapes of relaxing music in my car on the way into the office in the morning. Finally it dawned on me that this kind of music would be helpful to the patients and staff in the doctor's office where I work. I don't mean that elevator kind of music, but music that seems to go with the sounds and rhythms of nature.

Anne, another nurse joined in. "We have been using music in the labor and delivery rooms for quite a while now, and I think it has made quite a difference. Even when the situations get tense and a bit frantic, at least there's a rhythm to it all.

Some of the operating room personnel in our hospital are experimenting with playing different kinds of music as they work."

This gave Mark, a rehab counselor, an idea. "It might be worthwhile to ask the patients who are being operated on what kind of music is especially meaningful to them. I had a patient once, a young athlete who was in a coma from a car accident. His family knew that the theme music from "Chariots of Fire" had been especially meaningful to him as he was training for the Olympics. We played that music for him frequently while he was in the coma, and you could read on the monitors the dramatic, positive effect it had on his whole system."

"If we can find music that cools out the caregivers so we can concentrate on what we're doing for the patients," Ralph said, "the patients will gain from that as well."

WORKING IN A SELFCARING WAY

After arranging your work environment to support yourself and the kind of work you are doing there, the next question to ask yourself is "Am I working in a selfcaring way?" There is an African dialect in which the word for "*work*" is the same as the word for "*dance.*" Try asking yourself at the end of your work day, "How did the dance go today?"

There are other ways to tell if you have been working in a selfcaring way. Notice how much energy you have left for your own life at the end of the work day. Do you stumble home and immediately collapse into a sofa or bed? Are you too tired to eat? Or do you want to eat everything in sight, feeling the need for an energy transfusion? If staring at the T.V. is the extent of your off-duty recreation, you may need to give yourself a break through the way you are doing your work.

Viewing work as a dance, you might alter your rhythm and patterns of working. If work were a dance we would experience a variety of movements, faster segments followed by slower pauses and stops for rest. We would be pacing ourselves, focusing our energy on the specific steps at hand. There would be no such thing as "hurry up," and, rather than continually asking, "What's next?" we would experience the joy of celebrating our accomplishments.

SUPPORTIVE WORK FRIENDS

A family therapist, Carl Whitaker, recommends that everybody find what he calls a "cuddle group." This is a group of friends who accept you unconditionally and who meet solely for the purpose of supporting and celebrating each member. The more demanding and stress provoking your job, the more necessary the cuddle group.

The group can be as small as two people, as large as ten or twelve. It can be at the worksite. A woman colleague and I pledged to meet for dinner one evening a week when we both work late. Our commitment to one another helps us resist the urge to make one more phone call or catch up on paperwork. Instead, we take care of ourselves with nourishing food and conversation.

I know three men who refer to themselves as "cave buds". They check in with each other by phone during hectic work days. They support one another to take a work break for a golf game when their work schedules get especially demanding.

Another friend and I realized that, due to job changes, we would no longer see each other at work. To insure continued contact, we agreed to meet monthly for an extended lunch. We are considering inviting other caregivers to join what we call our "Sappy Social Workers' Support Group." We discuss our health, current work challenges, family crises — whatever is relevant. The main thing is that we, who are available for others at our work, can receive support for ourselves on a regular basis.

CREATING A SUPPORTIVE TEAM

Several years ago, as the world seemed to be tumbling down around my head careerwise, I got the opportunity to re-create my work life. A nurse/manager friend and her husband, a financial planner, led my husband and me in a career/life planning workshop. With flip chart and magic markers in hand, they encouraged us to dream and scheme our best-case work scenario. We developed a plan on paper, and, in only eight months, the actuality of a holistic mental health clinic was realized. We experienced for the first time the joys and struggles of designing with graph paper, making a business plan, and dealing with bankers, architects, accountants, and construction contractors. None of these were as difficult and time consuming as learning to build a collaborative work team. After much trial and error, we got far enough along in our own selfhealing to let go of what wasn't working in order to encourage and welcome people and things that did work.

We learned to say what we wanted but not to talk anyone into anything. We learned to consult with others, both staff and outside experts, and then to make the necessay decisions which were ours to make. And we learned to face the reality that we couldn't keep everybody happy all the time and take care of ourselves in the process.

We knew from the beginning the importance of recognizing and rewarding achievement and of celebrating personal and group accomplishments. It took practice learning to develop the following important attitudes:

1) Mistakes are natural events on the way to getting it right.

I knew an organization that gave an award for the most creative mistake of the month. Creative mistakes are celebrated because they demonstrate that the person is learning something new or discovering the need for improvements in the system. Too frequent mistakes on the job can signal the need for diversion or rest from the work task. Or frequent mistakes may mean an employee's personal stress is spilling over onto the work place.

2) Workers have personal lives and sometimes need time off from work to take care of family business.

We alternate emergency week-end coverage among professional staff so people can have holidays and weekends off while still seeing that the needs of clients are met. Offering access to counseling for support staff members going through family crises has paid off in increased work efficiency and/or the relocation of the employee to a different job assignment.

3) Work groups need practice in order to develop proficiency as a team.

Just because people know their own job doesn't mean they understand what the organization is trying to accomplish, what other staff members do or how to work together. Periodic staff retreats provide support staff, professionals, and consultants with the opportunity to get together in a relaxed environment to discover ways to work together and to learn the skills of collaboration.

4) A commitment to telling the truth is necessary for a supportive team to develop and grow through time.

As in our personal lives, in work teams we need to be able to work out differences and disagreements without blaming or shaming ourselves or others. We need to be able to show our vulnerabilities and allow others to show theirs as well. Continuing to pretend that everything is fine when it isn't or that we don't care when we do leads to a situation where we no longer care to stay in that workplace.

A staff member found the following item and posted it in the break room because she felt it was reflective of what we were trying to accomplish at our work place.

> **CELEBRATION POLICY**
>
> We publicly recognize achievements.
> We encourage spontaneous celebrations.
> We know that if we 're having fun,
> we work harder, smarter, and longer.
> We evaluate managers on their
> ability to create an environment in which
> it is a pleasure to work.
> Employees who spread gloom will be asked to leave.[5]

Signs For Your Office Wall

Since working in a selfcaring way involves what we tell ourselves and what we present to others, we can all use continual reminders of ways to take care of ourselves. As you decorate your work space, consider the following signs for your desk or office walls. You might invent your own friendly reminders for working in a selfcaring way.

> Celebrate each accomplishment
> in the moment, then
> Celebrate yourself
> in each moment.

> Work is not the way I earn my worth.

Sign for others:

> Your failure to meet your deadlines
> does not constitute an emergency for me.

(Your own special sign):

>

Consider the following prayer as a sign for your office wall. Or write your own and keep it handy to use when the going gets tough and you find yourself lost in paper work or peoplework.

Remind yourself, overdoing work can be too much of a good thing, damaging to health and well-being and a definite detriment to selfcare. When we get caught in this workaholism, we need to become selfhealing. Like people who overdo drinking or eating, we need help from our Higher Power. Try repeating the following prayer on a daily basis or write a prayer in your own words.

Prayer Of A Recovering Workaholic

May I do today the work which is truly mine to do
and support others in doing their duty as well.
May I take short breaks to catch my breath
and vary my tasks to prevent wearing myself out.
May I work with others in a partnership way,
celebrating all of our energies and talents.
May I communicate clearly my wants and needs
and listen to others from a receptive place of calm.
May I trust my efforts, however limited, will bring —
eventually — a positive outcome.
Allow me to feel finished at the end of each day.
May my relationship with time be a flowing duet.
                    Meanwhile,
          Help me to let go of my
             illusions of grandiose
                accomplishments,
          Of expecting of myself
             impossible feats.
          And, most especially,
          help me stop fighting
             the inevitable.

DOING YOUR WORK AS A DANCE

Now let's review and apply Psyche's skills of selfcaring to your work situation. This is an excellent way to ensure that your work is a dance celebrating your values, your gifts, and your abilities. The first step combines two of Psyche's skills, STEPPING BACK (4) and SORTING AND SEPARATING.(1)

   a) STEP BACK to gain a broader perspective and dream about your best-case work scenario. Next look at your current work environment and what is actually provided there. As you SORT AND SEPARATE your needs and values from what is actually provided in your work environment, you will gain information with which to EXERCISE CHOICE.(5)

b) Call on the help of supportive friends from inside and outside your work place. (PARTNERSHIP POWER (4))

c) If you determine that there are aspects of the work culture which interfere with your selfcare, work on LETTING GO (2) of whatever it is *you* do to cooperate with these forces. In the interest of your selfcaring, you may need to LET GO of potential promotions, specific financial rewards, or the prestige which comes from overworking and urging others to do likewise.

d) EXERCISE CHOICE (5) in the way you treat yourself. Make changes in aspects of your work environment that you have some say over. Alter your rhythm and patterns of working, allowing for variety, rest, and recovery. And don't forget to celebrate your efforts and accomplishments, even if others don't notice them.

NOTES

He who cannot dance
puts the blame on the floor.

Selfcare in a Large Organization 4

In legend there is relief from the enemy, sorrow is turned into gladness,
mourning into holiday. In life, only some of this is possible.
E.M.Broner, *A Weave of Women*

In addition to the physical aspects of one's environment (space,
furniture, color, sound, and light), many workplaces are also complex
social and organizational structures. Not simply an enactment of the
job descriptions and organizational flow charts, the work place culture
dictates behaviors, moods, and relationships. Many of the factors
which affect the culture of the work place are hidden from view.

Even though you have tended to the physical work environment,
established friends both inside and outside your work place, and
practiced doing your work as a dance, your selfcare is still not insured.

WORKING IN A DYSFUNCTIONAL ORGANIZATION

There are, proportionally, as many dysfunctional organizations
(corporations, governmental organizations, small businesses) as there
are dysfunctional families. And employees, like the children in a
dysfunctional family, often feel the negative effects of problems at the
executive level without knowing the story behind the scenes. Meet my
friend, Julie.

JULIE AND THE SINKING SHIP

It was early Saturday morning when I got the call. Julie
had just begun to figure out what had been happening to her at
the treatment center where she works. "I had been feeling
emotionally abused for some time, but after yesterday it seems
more like emotional rape, a betrayal by my supervisor," Julie
told me.

As we began to talk about her situation, Julie expressed a feeling of guilt for intruding on my personal time, especially since I hadn't heard from her in months. "I've been working 60 to 70 hours a week so I haven't had time for anything else lately," she said.

"I'm writing this morning on selfcare in the work place, and it sounds like your experiences are pretty relevant to my topic so, fire away!", I told her. "How did you happen to work such long hours?"

"I'm sure it's from a need to get the job done," Julie answered. "The turnover in staff has been incredible. I've been a therapist on the unit for a little over six months, and I've been there the longest. My original plan was to complete my thesis while I continued working. It finally became clear to me how impossible that plan was. I spoke to my supervisor last week asking for a leave of absence. He seemed supportive of the idea at the time, but after the way he attacked me at the meeting yesterday in front of the whole team — I don't know where he stands," Julie said.

After getting more details of the events of the last few months, the infighting among staff members, the discrepancy between what is said in private conversations and what happens in public meetings, and most of all, the splitting among staff members into "good parent/bad parent" roles in relation to the patients, I concluded, "You have a sick system and, just like a dysfunctional family, it's contagious to everyone in it."

"That's what I've been feeling, but what the staff says is that we are getting more seriously disturbed patients lately," Julie said.

"It's interactive," I said. "With the kind of staff turnover you've had, you're not providing a stable environment, and patients pick up and magnify the instability in the environment. One of my colleagues did biofeedback with patients in a treatment center for a number of years. She noted that she could always tell when an administrative change was in the process of occurring because the base line readings of all the patients in biofeedback therapy became higher than usual. And the readings for staff were even more elevated. This is hazardous work that we do, Julie, and staff can pick up the dis-eases of patients and administrators and add them to our own."

"This is what I am being accused of," Julie said. "There is one patient who is being scapegoated because he reacts to the environment. Whenever I take up for him, I become the scapegoat."

As we continued our telephone conversation, I glanced down at the manuscript in front of me, a page about the skills of selfcaring, and realized that Julie and I were moving through each of them. Julie began BUILDING AND USING PARTNERSHIP POWER when she reached out to me, overcoming her reticence to disturb my personal time. Together we began SORTING AND SEPARATING what part of her situation belongs to her and what belongs to others. Since I was an outsider to her specific situation but an insider to the kind of work she does and the type of facility where she works, we could STEP BACK together and see the big picture and the relationship of parts.

After Julie told me of her feelings of responsibility to her patients and their families, her concerns about her relationship to her supervisors, and her need to finish her degree, I told her, "I can put my advice to you into two words, Julie. Save yourself!"

As we talked about her LETTING GO and SURRENDERING in the face of overwhelming odds she said, "I'm beginning to feel a weight lifting from my shoulders."

"You really don't have the power to change this situation," I said. "You are not the captain, and you don't have to go down with the ship.

Use your power to save yourself, for yourself and for all the people you will be able to help once you complete your degree." I reminded her of her gifts and strengths and of the potential opportunities she could have EXERCISING CHOICE.

"Now I feel my heart opening, and I'm getting images of other possibilities as we speak," Julie said. As the conversation ended she said, "It really is all right to save myself, isn't it!"

Looking At Your Own Work Organization

As Julie's experience has so clearly illustrated, some work environments make selfcaring and selfhealing next to impossible, and attempting to take any action to change things may entail grave risk. But not taking action will have ramifications, too. Remembering our waltz of the flowers, staying in a situation which is unhealthy for plants and other living things could carry the greatest risk of all. Before you consider taking any action in your work place, take the following antidote to martyrdom. Repeat the following affirmation several times a day for at least three days before proceeding.

> **I am important. I am as precious and valuable as any one or all of my projects, goals, and achievements, and I matter as much as all my past, present, and future accomplishments.**

Working In A War Zone

In order to be able to take care of yourself at your work, you must first make sure that you are *not* working in a war zone. And selfcaring requires that if you are considering a job change, you make sure that the new work environment is a garden where you can blossom, not a war zone where you will be continually at risk. The following two checklists are offered for your consideration as you determine whether you are working in a war zone and, if so, how to survive such a situation.

How To Know If You Are Working In A War Zone

At first glance it would seem simple to determine if the organization where you work is operating as a war zone. In the case of open hostility, announced reorganizations, published threats of reprisal, and formal, confirmed notice of takeover attempt (both internal and external), *a state of war is quite clear.* However, by that time one or all of the following has probably already occurred:

a) You have been fired, or your boss has been fired which amounts to the same thing, though your demise may be slower.

b) Your best friend and colleague has been fired, so that all the fun and enjoyment has gone as you serve what seems like a life sentence, until retirement.

c) You have quit, landed on your feet at a place that doesn't seem any better than the last one, but they pay you more hush money.

One of the major goals of stress management is early identification of environmental stressors. "These boots were made for walking" is a refrain to sing while there is still breath left for singing and some spring left in one's gait. Becoming expert in managing stress (becoming selfcaring) means not going to the place of undue stress in the first place. Like the martial arts master who, sensing the energy of an approaching enemy, crosses the street and is not there when the enemy arrives.

To accomplish this slight-of-foot dance routine usually demands advanced skills of assessment, premonition, and more than a little inside information. It is in this spirit that the following advice is offered. (If you already know that your work place is in a war zone, see the next checklist below, "How To Be Selfcaring While Working In A War Zone.") If you are unclear about whether the work setting you are currently in or are considering entering is a war zone, continue reading.)

Ask yourself or someone currently working in the organization the following questions:

1. Do you feel like crying when you enter your office? If so, how many times a week does this occur? When you walk out of your office, does this feeling leave you? (Note: Due to early programming against crying, this will not be an accurate indicator for most men. Find a woman who works in the same environment and ask her this question.)
2. Do you feel like punching your fist through the wall of your office? How often does this feeling occur, and do you know any other people at the work site who are having this same experience? Note: Due to early and late messages of what constitutes lady-like behavior (socialization) this probably will not be an accurate indicator of most women's frustration. Ask a man these questions. Another method is to look around the work place at the faces of the men employed there and count how many of them *look* as though they feel like putting their fists through the wall and how many look as though they have already punched out a wall that day. Add these two numbers together and multiply by four. (This last operation is necessary due to men's socialization and continuing cultural practice of hiding their real feelings.)

If you have determined that you *are* working in a war zone, continue now to the next checklist.

How To Be Selfcaring While Working In A War Zone
1. First of all, realize — and never lose sight of the fact — that a war zone *is* where you are!
2. Set aside some specific time each day to plan your escape.
3. Take some time out each day to *escape* in your mind. Create pictures of peace and tranquility and nourish feelings of calm and serenity.

4. Move slowly and cautiously, and watch where you stand and step. Landmines are always hidden, and those left over from prior wars may be a surprise even to those who planted them.

5. Do not carry secret messages from one camp to another. This assumes you can tell who belongs to which army when everyone is dressed in civilian clothes. To be safe, do not carry or send any secret messages since intelligence, counter-intelligence, and counter-counter-intelligence operations are growth industries in war.

6. Develop connections with persons outside the war zone and with persons like yourself who work inside. Together create peace and tranquility as described above, and nourish and support one another. Only in extreme circumstances should you talk about the war, the soldiers, and their tactics or weapons.

7. In case you and your friends and colleagues have violated the above, perform a cleansing ritual. Forgive each other for causing each other pain, and then go rent a funny movie to watch together on your home video.

8. Should you or one of your friends get shot, observe the following steps in CPR (career-personality-rescue), otherwise the resulting wound to brain, personhood, and future life/work may be terminal.

   a) The first thing to do after you have been shot is to keep moving. You may be able to make it out of the war zone under cover of the cross-fire.

   b) Remove the bullet! As obvious as this step appears, many people have not done this. They have not allowed their wounds to heal. Present wars in work organizations often result when victims of prior wars do not remove old bullets and shrapnel.

   c) The removing of the bullet must be done in the presence of persons not involved in the war, or at the very least, in the presence of persons not afraid of blood, sweat, and tears. (As you may remember from watching reruns of the television show MASH, people who fire weapons on other humans are, by definition, afraid of blood, sweat, and tears.)

   d) Another tip from MASH — go ahead and bleed, sweat, and cry as long as you are not in the presence of enemies, for these biological responses are healthy and will aid in your healing.

9. Do not hurt or blame yourself for being in the war zone in the first place, for being wounded in the war (if that has been the case), or for bleeding from that wound. A great part of the world of work operates as a war zone. Although the war has not spread world-wide as yet, to find a work setting that is peaceful is more unusual than to find a government that spends no money on weapons.

10. Do not be surprised if some of your former friends and co-workers who must stay behind in the war zone are afraid to be seen with you. War zones, by their nature, operate with either/or battle slogans such as, "whose side are you on, anyhow," "all's fair in love and war," "if you aren't for me, you're against me!" and other such paranoid delusions. Don't play, even if it means losing some of your favorite playmates.

SOME FAR REACHING SOLUTIONS

After you have checked out the above possibilities and have made some of the changes in your physical environment suggested in the previous chapter, you may need to consider more far reaching solutions for taking care of yourself in the work place.

Selfcare in the work place is difficult (if not impossible) to maintain if you find yourself in certain types of situations. When your work is not having an effective outcome in spite of your best efforts, you are robbed of the good feelings which come from a job well done. Your workdays begin to feel as if you are rolling a large rock up a great hill, only to have it roll back down on you again. When you step back from the situation, you realize that the problems are not yours personally; they are at the level of the system. Here, the solutions are beyond what you can work out by yourself.

In some situations you can do your work and see an effective outcome, but in following the procedures and requirements of the job you injure yourself, your co-workers, or the people you are trying to serve. In these situations, selfcaring requires that changes be made *in the system* regarding how the job gets done, how it is funded, or how the caregivers and clients are treated in the process. Again, you are beyond what you can work out by yourself.

It's helpful to remember that performing the role of caregiver, whether professionally or personally, frequently leads to a recognition of the need for change at the system level. It's one thing to read about society's problems, it's another to deal with human needs closely and on a daily basis.

Sometimes this recognition of needs is overwhelming to the caregiver. Then selfcare for a "giver who cares" involves moving out beyond the immediate and personal to a larger arena. It definitely involves using partnership power as in the following examples:

- Parents of a retarded daughter are appalled by the lack of services for retarded persons in their state. They join other parents and begin identifying the desired programs. They form an organization and, through this vehicle, advocate for increased funds and services at the state and national level.

- Teachers and social workers providing services to pregnant teenagers identify the need for drug and alcohol education and treatment to prevent babies being born prematurely and addicted. The caregivers design a program and approach their local United Way organization for funding.

- Human service workers in a rural community, while continuing their own graduate education through a university extension program, identify a problem in the way local agencies serve (or fail to serve) minority persons. With assistance from their university professors and members of the minority communities, the caregivers write and carry out a grant which helps them design a system for delivering human services that works better.

- A mother loses a child when he is killed by a drunk driver. With other families in the same situation she forms an organization to lobby for more stringent laws and stronger enforcement in order to keep drunk drivers off the road. Public information campaigns help to enlighten communities so they no longer tolerate people driving while intoxicated.

Stories such as these could fill many volumes, as could the stories of caregivers in similar situations who were unable to transform their own pain. Some "givers who care" felt their situation hopeless and they became overwhelmed and unable to take action on their own or others behalf. Others attempted to change their world without fully realizing what they were up against, and in the process, didn't take the proper precautions to take care of themselves.

In order to deal with the natural result of being a caregiver — our enlightened understanding of how organizations and policies need to change in order to better meet human needs — we need a clearer understanding of how large systems work and how change can occur in them. I offer the following models for bringing about change and taking care of yourself in the process.

Creating Change At The System Level

As you contemplate change at the system level, keep in mind that the dance of selfcaring is not a solo or even a simple duet. Choreographing even small changes in large systems requires a cast of hundreds, including plenty of support from the audience. In addition, you must be extremely clear about what role you are playing and from which position and on what stage. Some maneuvers need to be accomplished from behind the scenes or in the wings, others from the next county, but always with a chorus of support.

No matter how gracefully introduced, any kind of change can generate a reaction of fear. And when money is involved, which is the most likely situation, people move into their survival mode instinctively. Some scenarios of change use the fear generated by a threat of taking money out of an organization to motivate people in the organization to allow particular changes to occur.

"Taking Money Out" Solutions

Though it may seem to you like scrip (paper money) in a Monopoly game, people in positions of power in large organizations become deadly serious about money coming in or out of their budgets.

Caregiving helper-types often avoid the Taking Money Out alternatives since the principal motivation is *fear*, not the preferred *doing the right thing*. But the fear of fines, reprisals, or lawsuits *can* move people to do the right thing. Then they can discover this new way of being is a reward in itself. Given the opportunity, people often come to realize how much fun it is to live and work in a garden where people and projects are busy blooming. Let's look at three scenarios which use the threat of taking money out of the organization.

It's The Law!

In the "It's The Law" scenario, the first step is to get a law, policy, or regulation enacted. Then quickly, while people still believe that the law will be enforced, help them to adhere to its requirements. Optimistically, this new way of doing things will be rewarding for everyone, and they will wonder how they ever got along in the old way. Working as a consultant to educators in school districts in Nebraska, I saw this solution work quickly and effectively.

In the mid-seventies, a small change was made in the language of the laws governing the operation of schools which received federal funds. Title IX stated that no school could discriminate on the basis of sex in any of their educational programs or policies.[1] The major effect was not on classroom schedules, textbooks, or teacher's salaries, though these issues were raised. The toughest question was "How can we have educational equity when we only have *one* gym?" Coaches and gym teachers spent many sleepless nights developing elaborate ways to give the girls access to the gymnasium for their sports without interfering with the boys' sports schedule.

One administrator was the father of four daughters, and seeing the situation from the girls' perspective helped him understand the intent of the new law. He turned down proposals which gave the girls the gym between 5 a.m. and 7 a.m. before school and on Sundays during church services.

"Let's put it this way," he said; "The girls can have the gym Monday, Wednesday and Friday after school one week, and then after school Tuesday and Thursday the following week. Or, the girls and boys can alternate the use of the gym after school; one week the boys have it, the next week it's the girls turn. Or, if you don't like any of these ideas we can do it this way: The girls can have the gym all to themselves for the next 50 years, since the boys have had it totally to themselves for the last 50!"

So, since nobody could figure out how to prevent it, the girls were given the opportunity to play sports. The outcome of this experiment was that the girls liked to play sports just like their brothers and gained the same value from the experience that boys had always gained. (They developed healthy bodies and strong minds, and practiced being team players.) As it turned out, many parents had daughters as well as sons, and they came to the games and supported the school for their daughters' sake, just as they had done for their sons. And people discovered that the honor of the school, the village or town, and the state could be defended by the girls as well as by the boys. It became just as much fun for "our girls to beat their girls" as it was for "our boys to beat their boys."

Eventually, it became fun to *do the right thing*. As one principal of a small school district said in response to being told what a good job his school had done opening opportunities for girls, "We are American citizens here," he exclaimed with great pride. "We obey the law!"[2]

LET'S STRIKE!

A second scenario comes from the strategies of labor unions. Millions of workers in America have used collective bargaining and negotiations, sometimes involving the threat or actual use of strikes to achieve better working conditions, salaries, and other benefits. But caregivers have shied away from these approaches, continuing quietly to provide services for others without thought for ourselves. This selfless "I'm not doing this for the money" attitude has resulted in caregivers appearing as *saps* and having the work they do less valued than occupations that demand higher pay.

On those rare occasions when caregivers *have* used collective bargaining and negotiation (teachers and nurses striking, for example), the results were often an improvement in service. Smaller classroom size, while improving working conditions for teachers, also means each child can receive more attention from his/her teacher. Higher pay for nurses encourages more young people to consider a nursing career and alleviates the shortage of nurses.

A selfcaring approach to these issues is for everyone to win, but those who live in the power-over-others model don't always view it that way. There is great danger that the people in power will regard your interest in improving services and in taking care of yourself as a declaration of war. You would then be working in a war zone with only one move left: to plan your immediate escape.

On the other hand, it may be possible to bargain and negotiate changes which benefit yourself, your colleagues, and your clients without starting a war. You will need to sing the song of your request in the largest chorus you can organize. Enlist singers from outside the organization to perform featured solo roles, highlighting the beauty and wisdom of your choir's major themes. Finally, connect this all up with everyone's funny bone, so that even if the situation becomes hopeless, it will not be considered too serious.

My Lawyer Can Beat Up Your Lawyer

The third scenario in the Taking Money Out solution involves litigation or the threat of litigation. This strategy can be combined with other versions of taking money out mentioned above. Civil rights activists, for example, employed collective action by disobeying the law in order to get unjust laws changed. This was frequently combined with a class action suit where a lawsuit was filed on behalf of all the people affected by an organization's policies or practices.

WARNING: Due to the tendency of organizations to move quickly from a garden-like state to a state of war; litigation and threat of same should only be done from outside the organization, preferably from outside of the state or territory involved. This way, progress in human consciousness can occur without the sacrifice and painful death of the person who first thinks up or stands up for each new great idea.

FURTHER TIPS

• Taking Money Out solutions do not represent a quick fix unless the organization, through its Risk Management Department, decides it is *the right thing* to avoid expensive court costs. Settling out of court will still probably mean that if you are the person who started all of this you need to leave the organization. You will be seen as a *trouble maker*, even by many of the people who are benefiting from the changes you helped to bring about. You will only get satisfaction if you are able to see yourself, as Bernie Seigel suggests, as being used for a purpose, recognized by yourself, as mighty.

• If you and your friends get involved in a court case as a way of Taking Money Out to educate the organization, you must plan on living an unusually long life. This will be necessary in order to find out how it turns out. Usually by the time these cases come to a hearing, no living person on either side has any memory, personally (or through family oral histories and genealogies), of what the case was about.[3]

• If the people in the organization respond to your Taking Money Out solution as a declaration of war (and this is highly likely), do not be surprised by the treachery which will follow. As a caring helper-type, your consciousness is ever aware of the importance of relationships and the connection of all living things. It is hard for you to fathom the potential wartime posture and attitude which can be ignited at a seemingly small provocation. This "All Bets Are Off, Never Mind What I Said Yesterday/All's Fair In War/Get Them Before You Get Gotten" attitude creates, at the very least, extreme confusion. Just because you do not feel that what you have done is an act of war, either declared or undeclared, does not mean that the other folks are not defining the situation as war.

Some experts feel that the move to define differences of opinion as acts of war is merely an excuse for some "power-over" types to justify stepping outside the bounds of human decency. This no-holds-barred approach means that the rule book is out the window, no referee is present for the contest, and you must run (not walk) to the nearest place of shelter. Do not regard leaving the field as an act of cowardice but rather as an act of loving selfcare. Remember, saving one's face while losing the rest of one's body/mind is no victory at all.

"PREVENTING MONEY BEING TAKEN OUT" SOLUTION

In the following story you will see how sometimes, just keeping the programs and funds we have can be a glorious victory for "givers who care". This strategy down plays the role of fear, although elected officials are always aware of the upcoming election and the voters they must be accountable to.

A Peaceful Piece Of The Pie

Once upon a time a particular state legislature was facing a particularly serious budget deficit. Having at one time *done the right thing* for education, roads, and welfare services, they were casting about for places to cut spending rather than raise revenue. Most politicians are convinced that if they raise taxes, they lower the boom on their own political careers. So remember, they need lots of help to avoid an overwhelming fear of their own annihilation while they are *doing the right thing*.

Among the programs and items the legislator had slated for elimination were three advocacy organizations, the Mexican-American, Native American, and Women's Commissions. Although these programs were small and cutting them wouldn't save the state very much money, they were seen as easy targets since they were run by caring helper-types for the benefit of people who had little power or influence in the first place.

A peaceful campaign was organized involving as many people from both inside and outside the organizations as possible. They were to sing the song,"Save The Commissions" to the tune of "Give Me Some Men Who Are Stout-Hearted Men." The women from all three commissions did what women of all cultures do when the going gets tough. They went immediately to their kitchens and began baking. On the morning of the final deliberations, in the great hall where all great deliberations take place, on each legislator's desk was an appetizing pie. In the center of each pie was a fork with a small flag attached. The message on the flag read: "We don't want the whole pie; we are just asking for our own little piece, 1/10 th of 1 % of the state budget. Fork it over, fellas!"

And the people of the land won, living to fight peacefully another day. Truth, Justice, and the American Way demand an ever continuing and expanding sense of vigilance, along with a continually developing sense of humor.

So much for Taking Money Out or Preventing Money From Being Taken Out solutions. In the Monopoly game of making changes in large organizations you might consider the positive strategies of bringing money into the organization.

"Bringing Money In" Solutions

Let's say you have some great ideas about how services could be improved in your organization. Nobody has any problem with the idea; there just aren't enough resources, especially money, to carry it out. Here is where the Bringing Money In solution can be helpful. Included in this solution are such strategies as writing grants for special projects, raising funds from sources which don't normally contribute to your organization, or designing ways for the organization to make money and/or receive prestige from something that means *doing the right thing*.

FALLACIES IN "THE BRINGING MONEY IN" SOLUTIONS

The Bringing Money In approach to change in an organization is not as dangerous to your personhood or job tenure as the Taking Money Out scenarios. But there are fallacies which can interfere with your being able to use this Bringing Money In solution.

Fallacy 1: People in the organization must salute and pledge allegiance to the goals of your projects in order for the project to be successful.

As we saw in the Take Money Out solutions, people may not understand or realize how satisfying it is going to be to help the sick, wounded, and needy or to eliminate, through preventive programs, the need for such help. If the people who run your organization had the same awareness as you have, there probably would be no need for you to come up with your ideas in the first place. The world itself would be a significantly different place. The best you can hope for is that people in your organization will ignore you benignly and let you work to accomplish your goals.

Fallacy 2: People at the top need to have your value system in order for the projects to work out.

Just like the politicians who want to be re-elected, your bosses want to hold on to their positions, enhance their reputations, and bloom where they are planted. If what you want to do can be seen as meeting *their* goals you have a chance, especially if you are bringing in or generating the money yourself.

In the beginning it helps if the source of the money brings with it some prestige for your boss and/or organization. One way to remember this is that "some money is gold, not just the usual green stuff." People and organizations who give away money (Fancy Friends From Afar) know this, and you need to proceed with caution so as not to be hurt by their good intentions. Outside funding sources have a tendency to under-fund with the green stuff, relying on the "golden halo" effect of their money to open doors for the project. Level with your Friends From Afar about what you are really up against in your organization. Otherwise the demonstration project ends up demonstrating what a lot of people have been thinking all along. (It's better to keep things the way they are.)

Fallacy 3: Your organization's commitment to the changes will endure after the money is no longer coming in.

Enduring commitment is the best-case scenario, but it is improbable if the project has been of short duration. Also, the loss of funds may be interpreted as a loss of face by the organization's leaders. People in organizations *can* become what they do, but only if they are kept saluting, pledging allegiance, and applauding *doing the right thing* long enough for the memory traces to take hold in their body/minds.

"NOT-ONE-RED-CENT" SOLUTION

This third solution to becoming and remaining selfcaring while making changes in large organizations I have called the "Not-One-Red-Cent" solution. In this scenario you spend time in a work organization, learning all you can from the experiences provided. You take special precautions, in the best selfcaring tradition, to avoid being fatally wounded in war zones. You move up in the corporation as far as the system will allow. You learn all you can and then you leave, taking with you all that you have learned to set up your own organization. The real fun comes when you bid against your former organization as an independent contractor, and you win the contract.

You can take pleasure in this solution for, not only are you now free to *do your own right thing* in your own caring helper way, but you can delight in the fact that the organization which drove you out will get *not-one-red-cent* of the rewards you are now able to earn through your knowledge and abilities.

MOVING ON

Many caregivers get caught up in the treacherous maze of organizational politics. Feeling that our cause is just, our values are right, or that the need is so great, we forget to protect ourselves so that we may live to fight another day. Like Julie, the mental health professional who worked 60 hours a week, we need to realize it is OK to save ourselves. And saving ourselves involves recognizing the true reality of what we are up against.

Consult with your "Cuddle Group" or "Cave Buds" and other support persons, both inside and outside your organization, to be sure you are seeing the situation with clarity. Determine whether the scenarios for making changes in your organization (described above) are feasible in your situation. If making changes is not feasible (and you have done what you can to get people in the organization to address the issues) perhaps the time for letting go of your work situation has arrived. You need to let go of your work situation if the following conditions exist in your work place:

- The person in direct line of authority over you is an addict and is making work decisions out of his or her disease. (Your boss is a practicing alcoholic or workaholic and expecting everyone who works for him/her to do and see things as he/she does.)

- You are given an impossible job without the resources to accomplish it. (Funding or staff levels are so low you have determined you are doing more harm than good to yourself and/or clients.)

- The organization has changed priorities, moving away from the mission and function of your job. (You find it too painful to stand by and watch your project dismantled.)

- You are being required to go against your own core values. (Helping people to stay in damaging situations creates internal stress for you.)

- The meaning of your life can only be lived by moving on to your next work challenge. (Sometimes we outgrow our jobs. Even if we work in a healthy organization, the right step in our own selfcaring can be letting go without malice or rejection.)

Letting go of a job can be as difficult as letting go of anything else we put our hearts and minds into. Most of us rely on our jobs for financial security and physical survival, not to mention meeting our needs for achievement and expression of ourselves. This codependence on our jobs means that we need a lot of help in being able to be selfcaring and selfhealing in the work place.

Sometimes moving away from a work situation which is not selfcaring means learning to have faith that the values we hold are connected to something greater than ourselves. Rather than seeing ourselves as isolated voices in the wilderness, we need to experience connection.

One of the newest of the support groups (based on the twelve steps of Alcoholics Anonymous) is one for people in the helping professions. Codependents Anonymous for Helping Professionals (CODAHP) assists people whose jobs involve helping and serving others with their own selfcare. These groups, like all the twelve step groups, help members to recognize their powerlessness to control others, and they encourage the development of a perspective which includes relationship to a larger order or Higher Power.[4]

Whatever resources you choose, whatever scenarios of change you decide to pursue — keep reminding yourself of the following:

> **I am as valuable as any and all of my projects, goals, and accomplishments, and as such I am deserving of having my needs met as I perform my life work.**

A time to weep and a time to laugh,
a time to mourn and a time to dance.

A Selfcaring Home Life

5

In the sense in which a man can ever be said to be at home in the world,
he is at home not through dominating, or explaining, or appreciating,
but through caring and being cared for...
Milton Mayeroff, *On Caring*

As the sun fades slowly in the West, the end of another workday
is at hand. Following your footsteps down the hall to the street, the
Muzak melody strums, "Oh, give me a home where the buffalo roam..."
You begin to sing along... "Where seldom is heard a discouraging
word, and the sky is not cloudy all day."

That's entertainment, but it's not even remotely connected to the
reality of most peopleworkers' lives. The following list describes
scenes which may be a bit more familiar.

a) You haven't seen the sun in weeks, and that's not because
it's the rainy season in Seattle. Since your job involves
serving others, you must be available to them when they
want you. Many clients, patients, and customers want
services before or after their own work day. Of course,
their wish is your command, so you are available before
the sun is up and long after the sun has gone down.

b) There is no such thing as being off duty. You wear a
beeper at your belt and know that at any time of the day
or night your life may be interrupted. Like a cowboy on
night watch, you rest and try to sleep with one ear attuned
to the coyote's howl.

c) You go home, but you carry your not-so-brief case full of
paperwork which needs to be done before dawn. Your
family has more than a few discouraging words to say
about your requests to be left alone or to be excused from
household chores for the evening.

d) You go home, leaving your work at work, and begin struggling through your second job on *that* "range." This "moonlighting" means a different arena for the same caring, helping role.

e) Or, you can't go home because you are already there. After being the home caregiver all day, you must now keep yourself from strangling the person you live with who is playing out one of the scenarios above.

There are many different versions of the caregivers' homecoming, but the themes are quite similar. Too much work and not enough play. Too much taking care of others and not enough time for oneself. What is the particular theme song that expresses *your* home lifestyle?

"As Long As He Needs Me" (I know ....)

"All Of Me" (why not take ....?)

"Only The Lonely"

"Hard Day's Night " (and I've been working like.......)

"Sixteen Tons (..........................Another day older and...")

"I'm Late, I'm Late (for a very important date.")

(Here name your favorite_____.)

Whatever your particular verse and chorus, for those of us who do caring work, protecting personal time while meeting family responsibilities provides the supreme challenge to our ability to take care of ourselves.

THE ENDLESSNESS OF A CARING LIFESTYLE

In our personal and family life, those of us who do caring work for a living may feel that our work is never finished. There is no such thing as time out or time off, even for very good behavior. When we are operating from a selfless "don't think of yourself, do for others" frame of reference, we are in danger of burning out from too much of a good thing. In relating to family and friends, we are presented hourly with opportunities for losing ourselves in the clamor of others' needs. And having "given at the office," we may have little left to give ourselves as we respond to the demands of others at home.

Laura, a working mother with young children, describes it this way: "I have an image of myself as a bass cello with strings running up and down the front of me from my head to my feet. Other people can't see the strings, and even I don't know they are there. Only my children know about these magic strings. Whenever they want something from me, they just reach over near my heart, and pluck a string. They know just which one will cause me to vibrate, which one will get the response they want from me."

Since it is part and parcel of our lifestyle to live in caring connection to others, we cannot hope to run out of relatives. When children grow up, parents grow old, and there are still plenty of people who will pluck our strings if we let them.

Valerie has raised four children. Now she comes home to her husband's mother who has been living with them for the past year. "It was supposed to be temporary, but now I'm beginning to wonder if this is a permanent arrangement. Bill's mom came because she was recovering from hip surgery and couldn't stay alone. Just when she got over that, she got a case of the shingles. Now she's broken her ankle, and I'm afraid to go home from work and find out what's happened next. Bill travels a great deal, so most of the caregiving in this situation is falling to me. I'm truly sorry for all her misfortune, but she doesn't treat me well, and I wish she wouldn't take her misfortune out on me."

Building Boundaries

So what are we to do about the difficult dilemma of taking care of ourselves in the face of myriad requests from those we love, from those who are depending on us? As family members, we need each other and rely on one another. But sometimes the burden of responsibility isn't shared evenly, according to each person's age and ability. Sometimes we overdo our doing for others which interferes with their doing for themselves and developing their own selfcaring skills.

Selfcaring and selfhealing in our families means that we each take responsibility for ourselves, creating strong boundaries between ourselves and those we love. Let's review the skills of selfcaring and look at them from a family perspective.

The first one, SORTING AND SEPARATING means that each family member is seen as an individual. Children are not simply extensions of their parents but are encouraged to identify and express their own needs and wants. Parents are not just extensions of the families in which they grew up. Each partner in the marriage works to resolve her/his individual issues with the family of origin. Continuing the sorting and separating of individual and family issues from their current relationship enables the couple relationship to uniquely meet the needs of the two people creating it.

As we relate to growing children, sorting and separating is a continuous process. We begin by doing everything for an infant and gradually through the years transfer responsibilities for selfcaring to the growing child. Since the way parents handle things has such a strong impact on children, we parents, particularly women, get in the habit of asking ourselves when children have difficulties, "What have I done wrong?"

When one of my sons had difficulty learning to read I questioned whether I had nursed him too long or too little, whether I had prepared him properly for the birth of his younger brother, or whether I needed to help him more with his homework. This parental dedication is admirable, but we must continually sort and separate what rightly belongs to us regarding our children's behavior, and guard against taking on what rightly belongs to the child, the school, or the community.

LETTING GO AND SURRENDERING means allowing each family member to make her/his own mistakes and hold his/her own opinions. Letting go of control over others means not interfering with somebody else's business.

Sometimes marriage partners have an unspoken (and, I believe, unhealthy) pact in which they attempt to take care of each other. This isn't just a division of labor in which one person performs certain chores like taking care of the cars or household finances, while the other does the shopping or cooking. Most organizations, families included, need some division of labor. And in circumstances of illness or injury, we do need to be cared for until we can get back on our own feet. But when one able bodied adult is taken care of by another, this is an act of boundary violation and interferes with that person's caring for him/herself.

In considering the above statements, we are already moving to the third selfcaring skill, BUILDING and USING PARTNERSHIP POWER. One of the most difficult experiences in life is to be in a relationship with someone you love who is not taking care of him/herself. In fact, it is important to note here: *Do not attempt to build partnership power* with someone who is not committed to taking care of him/herself. This would be similar to jumping into deep water to save someone who is drowning when you don't know how to swim. Nothing is gained when both people go down. Families can be mutual benefit societies when all members are committed to taking care of themselves and assisting each other.

So the power struggles we are all familiar with in families can be eliminated. Instead of Mom saying, "How can I get my son up early enough to get to school on time?" she says, "Son, how can I be helpful to you in your getting up early enough to get to school on time?"

STEPPING BACK to see the big picture and the relationship between parts is essential when we find ourselves getting caught in somebody else's business. As one mother whose daughter has had problems with drug addiction told me, "When I find the effects of my daughter's actions coming back on me, I'm standing too close. It's time to back up and get out of the way." And of course, depending on how self-destructive the daughter's behavior is, the mother may need to be in the next county for her own protection.

Selfcaring and selfhealing in intimate relationships require that we step back and observe ourselves in the act of doing whatever it is we and other family members are doing. We are each a part of whatever pattern is going on, and we are EXERCISING CHOICE only if we can identify what we are doing. STEPPING BACK gives us the opportunity to gain this important perspective.

The ability to SAY NO and YES in EXERCISING CHOICE grows out of the other skills. For most caregivers, saying yes to ourselves and no to others takes practice and more than a little courage.

FRIENDS AND LOVERS: A HEALTHY PACT

So what does a healthy pact between adults look like? Consider the following:

I RECOGNIZE MY RIGHT AND RESPONSIBILITY
TO TAKE CARE OF MYSELF.

I RECOGNIZE AND RESPECT YOUR RIGHT AND RESPONSIBILITY
TO TAKE CARE OF YOURSELF.

I PLEDGE TO MAKE MY OWN SELFCARING
A PRIORITY IN MY LIFE AND ASK THAT YOU MAKE YOUR OWN SELFCARING A
PRIORITY IN YOURS.

I PLEDGE TO DO WHATEVER I CAN
TO ASSIST YOU IN TAKING CARE OF YOURSELF
AND ASK THAT YOU DO THE SAME FOR ME.

I PROMISE TO ASK FOR YOUR HELP IN MY TAKING CARE OF MYSELF
WHEN I FEEL THE NEED FOR SUCH HELP. I WOULD LIKE
YOU TO ASK FOR MY HELP WHEN YOU FEEL THE NEED FOR IT.

WE BOTH UNDERSTAND THAT OUR RELATIONSHIP IS BASED
ON EACH OF US TAKING CARE OF OURSELVES.
WHEN EACH OF US ACTS OUT OF WHAT IS TRULY BEST FOR US,
IT RESULTS IN WHAT IS BEST FOR THE RELATIONSHIP
AND FOR EACH OF US AS INDIVIDUALS AS WELL.

DOUBLE AND TRIPLE WHAMMIES[1]

Double and triple whammies are what I call the compounding of misfortune when we aren't taking care of ourselves in relation to those we love, or when we are too closely involved with someone who isn't taking care of him/herself. The effects of a slip, a fall, or a mistake are doubled or tripled when family members are holding on to each other too tightly. Do you recognize yourself and/or your family members in the Double Whammies below?

Love/Hate

I love you more than life itself.
You hate yourself
for not being able to respond to me.
I am hurt by your mistreatment of yourself.
I provoke you to mistreat me instead.
You are hurt by seeing the hurt
you inflict on me.

The Chase

You run from yourself.
I run after you.
You see yourself in me.
You run further from me.
Now you are lost from yourself,
And from me.

Despair

You hurt me.
I think I must have
done something wrong
For you to hurt me so.
I take what you send out,
Sharpen it as a dagger,
And run myself through.
You blame me for bleeding.
And I blame myself for ever
having loved,
for being vulnerable,
for having been born,
for being me.

Take some time to construct your own whammies. Here's how.

1) Begin with some behavior that you don't like in another person.
2) Add a line that describes your response
3 And then a line for his/her response, until the entire pattern is complete.
4) You are on the right track if you notice that the pattern is a circle and begins to repeat itself.

Now go back and identify a place in the cycle where you can EXERCISE CHOICE. See what other selfcaring skills you can use: LETTING GO AND SURRENDERING as you give another back the responsibility for his/her own life; SORTING AND SEPARATING what is yours and what belongs to the other person; BACKING AWAY further, or getting some help (PARTNERSHIP POWER) from outside the family system.

COMBINING THE SELFCARING SKILLS

As important as each one of the skills of selfcaring are, they rarely are used in isolation. It can be nearly impossible, for example, to *say no* to someone in your personal life if you have not done your own sorting work. And once caught in a power struggle, you may need some help (*partnership power*) in *standing back* for a clear perspective. And selfcaring can be nearly impossible if you have not healed from early conditioning about yourself and about how you are *"supposed"* to be in the world. Let's look now at a case example of the interconnection of selfcaring skills with selfhealing in a story of one woman's successful healing from her childhood traumas.

THE WAVE

Meet Joan, an attractive, slender woman in her early thirties. Professionally Joan had achieved success and a regional reputation in the human relations field with her writing, consulting, and training activities. But her personal life had become so difficult that she had come to dread time off, and often she overworked in order to avoid dealing with friends and family. Especially with male friends, Joan had difficulty knowing what she wanted and being able to stick with her own agenda in the face of a friend's requests. At the time we began her individual therapy Joan was feeling torn between two male friends, both of whom seemed to want "all of her."

"When I am talking with Bob, even on the phone, I begin to feel trapped, like I am suffocating." While Joan described her emotional symptoms, she gestured to her upper chest, indicating this as the place in her body where she feels the pressure.

"The more he seems to be pressuring me to spend time with him, the more uncomfortable I feel. As time goes on, I lose touch with what I am feeling and so I don't stand up for what I want because I don't even know what that is."

Joan's healing work over several weeks developed a clearer awareness of what she does physically to inhibit her breathing and when this inhibition occurs in her relationships with her male friends. After stepping back and looking at her pattern, Joan told the women in her therapy group, "It seems crazy, but it's like I feel I have to respond to whoever needs me the most." The women in the group nodded agreement with Joan's discovery since they too were often unduly affected by other peoples' expressions of need for them. Group members laughed and teased one another good-naturedly about this helping habit. As one woman put it, "This system could lead to developing some pretty pitiful friends, each vying for the 'neediest-of-the-week award'."

Over a period of several months Joan endeavored to interrupt this "fright and flight" response reaction she had whenever friends wanted something from her. Recognizing that everything is connected physically, emotionally, mentally, and spiritually, Joan embarked on a multifaceted program for her own selfcaring and selfhealing. She began taking lessons in karate even though she couldn't imagine "hurting someone on purpose." She continued working individually and in a group with me as her therapist. In her imagination she practiced developing a relaxation response and relating to her friends from a place of comfort and centeredness within herself. And, in her real life with friends, there were gains and improvements in her ability to sort out what she wanted from what others expected from her.

After about nine months of concerted effort, Joan hit a place of deep discouragement. "I feel as though I've come so far in my healing, yet not far enough," Joan told me. "It's almost like I'm afraid for things to go too well, like I'm waiting for the next wave of bad feelings to hit."

Picking up on Joan's metaphor, I said, "So, whenever you venture away from the beach and into the water, waves come along to push you back up on the shore?"

"Yes, and the more progress I make, the more violent the

waves seem. I'm not sure I can stand up to them," Joan said with more than a touch of discouragement in her voice.

Joan lay on her back on the massage table for her Rubenfeld Synergy^2 session with me. Using the suggestions of my gentle touch and her own creative imagery, she moved quickly to a now familiar place of peace and rest.

"So, where is that wave now?" I asked her.

"It feels like it's suspended over my head, waiting to come down on me when I least expect it," Joan said, gesturing above her right shoulder.

"So it sneaks up on you. Well, what does the wave want from you? What is it trying to say to you?" I asked.

Joan's face grew pale, and terror built in her eyes as she responded to the questions with strong emotion, "It says, '*You are bad! You are bad! You are bad!*' "

In a voice of gentle indignation I probed her "wave" further. "What did she do that is so bad? Does she get to know what she did, to know of what she is accused?"

Speaking as the wave, Joan answered in an accusing voice, "You don't meet the standards."

"Well, that's a different story," I said, expressing some excitement and relief. "Not meeting the standards? Is that it? Well, that's different. Do we get to know whose standards you aren't meeting? Just for the record?"

"The standards of my family, the Chaplin family standards!" Joan said with a look of surprise that the information came from her, as she did not know she knew it until that moment.

Joan's family had instilled in her many of the common messages which keep people from feeling good about themselves. Joan was given unrealistic standards, standards that would have been unrealistic whatever her age and skill level. Perfection was the minimum standard in the household where she grew up. She was expected to be perfect or at least to suppress her own needs and wants and "act like" she was perfect. She was expected to be strong and take care of her parents and always try to please the adults in her life.

In addition to all this, in her adult life, she felt the need to hurry through her days and weeks, continuing to try harder to meet these impossible standards, and continuing to feel bad about herself for falling short of the mark.

After her discovery of how these feelings and ideas were programmed into her system, Joan's next steps included sorting and examining which standards and traditions from her family of origin she wanted to continue to observe and live up to and which to let go of. Freeing the energy and tension she was using to keep the "wave" at bay meant that her images in therapy changed along with her relationships in real life. A short time later she pictured herself swimming in deep, clear water and sending the following message to her male friends about the type of partnership power she wants in her close relationships.

"I enjoy swimming with you, but I won't be holding you up any more! I plan to be swimming in deep water far from shore. I'd rather swim alone than swim in the deep with someone who isn't a strong swimmer and cannot hold his own when the water is over his head!"

Developing Your Own Standards

Many caregivers have been given messages similar to Joan's. Do you have some or all of the following? "Be Perfect!" "Be Strong!" "Try Harder!" "Please others!" And "Hurry up!" (in complying with all the other messages).[3] Becoming selfcaring means we must undo or redo these messages. And it's helpful to get hints from others about how they can feel comfortable with their home lives.

Caregivers' Creative Solutions

Marie, a social worker and agency executive told me, "I'm pretty greedy for life, so I knew if I wanted to have it all, I'd have to get some help. My husband and I are quite a team, and we've been training our two kids to be a part of the team as well."

"Taking turns," "teamwork," and "cooperation" were frequently used words I heard when interviewing successful career women who also felt some measure of satisfaction with their home lives.

"We all pitch in and clean the house on Saturday mornings, and then we can go to a movie or do something else fun in the afternoon," Coleen, a bank teller told me. "Before we organized things in this way, I dreaded facing the weekend and all I had to do at home while my colleagues who didn't have children were celebrating, 'Thank God It's Friday.'"

Getting meals on the table presented the most challenging family task and also the most creative solutions from the women I interviewed.

When Karen, a policewoman, married her second husband, combining her two children with his three, she reported nearly "coming unglued" until they figured out a strategy for mealtime.

"My husband works at a treatment center, and we borrowed the system used there. We held a "community meeting" to plan and carry out a system which would be fair to everybody in the family, instead of having me do it all, which was my first approach. Now my husband and I each cook dinner one night a week. Each of the older kids takes a night, and we have one night we call "sandwich night" when the younger kids are in charge. One night is fast food night, so this makes it all manageable. Each cook takes responsibility for planning his/her own meals and making sure the supplies they need get on the grocery list. Now there's time for me to relax in the evening and even help the kids with their homework."

A "casserole co-op" was another creative strategy I heard about. In this model, three families each make one special meal over the week-end. They triple the recipe, and on Monday the families trade the extra portions with each other. In order for this to work, family size needs to be fairly compatible and food allergies and preferences similar. It's a great way to get your kitchen labor to go far and come back to you with an extra measure.

I gleaned some additional suggestions from the women for taking care of themselves in their home places.

"Lower your standards, " advised Shirley. "When we expect our homes to be perfectly tidy and perfectly clean we set ourselves up to feel bad about ourselves most of the time. Or if we do achieve these unreal standards, the quality of our family life suffers because everybody feels afraid to really live in the house."

"Simplify! Simplify! is my motto," Helen, a woman minister said. "I ask myself, 'do I need these clothes, these extra utensils? What can I eliminate so I won't have to take care of it or find a place for it?' Seems like at first we own things, and then, if we're not careful, our things own us."

"One of my favorite strategies for taking care of myself at home is to celebrate often," said Lois, the mother of three. "Being together as a family isn't just about getting the work done and getting the kids to do their homework. What I remember from my childhood were the fun times, the celebrations, the rituals of birthdays and holidays, and planning vacations. If we're overdoing work, whether at home or at the office, we don't have time or energy for these joyful events."

THE IMPORTANCE OF FRIENDS

Family members, with the exception of spouses, are in our lives by chance and not by choice. Relatives are thrust upon us by the circumstances of our birth, while friends are a different matter. Friends are freely chosen and can be some of the greatest resources for our own selfcaring. Since they want what is truly best for us, friends encourage and assist us in taking care of ourselves. Friends don't expect us to be perfect, and, seeing our wounds, they offer encouragement for our healing. Friends believe in us through times of self doubt. They offer friendly support when the world seems unfriendly. Friends appreciate the honor of being a friend and celebrate our friendship as a gift to their lives.

Some people are fortunate to be able to continue the friendships of their childhood and youth into their adult lives, but most of us have moved far away (either physically, mentally, or emotionally) from early relationships. And many of us are too busy with our caring, helping responsibilities at work and at home to nurture and develop true adult friendships. Circumstances in our current culture have not made it easy to locate persons who are good candidates for friendships.

WANTED: GROWNUP FRIENDS

Song: "Where Have All The Grown-ups Gone?"
(sung to the tune of "Where Have All The Flowers Gone?")

Where have all the grown-ups gone? long time passing,
Where have all the grown-ups gone long time ago.
Where have all the grown-ups gone?
* Gone to grave yards, everyone,
When will we ever learn?
When will we ever learn?

Subsequent verses:

* Climbed into bottles, everyone,	** Taking pills, everyone,*
* Drowned in drugs, everyone,	** Hooked on sex, everyone,*
* Lost in work, everyone,	** Hiding in food, everyone.*

THE JOY OF TRUE GROWNUP FRIENDS

A number of years ago Margaret Mead warned the world that there were too many children for the number of adults who were caring for them. As a person who cares, helps, and gives to others in your work life and then repeats the same patterns in your home life, you would probably join me in telling Margaret, "It's worse than even you had predicted."

It's not just the number of real, genuine, bona fide children. Actually, they can be a true joy and relief from the pseudo-kids who have passed the age of legal majority without coming close to real adulthood. If you are a person who cares for others at work and home, you need friends in your off-duty life who are true grown-ups. As you seek out such persons, consider asking yourself the following questions.

• •

THE TEST FOR A TRUE GROWNUP

1. Is this person big enough to come out and play with you! If he/she needs permission from someone else (mother, father, or former spouse), then he/she is not grownup enough for you. This also applies to persons who need pills, drugs, and other chemicals in order to play and have a good time. They most definitely are not grownup enough to be a true friend.
2. Is this person old enough to play alone and keep entertained when you are busy elsewhere? If you have to be the social director, travel agent, and hostess with the mostest for your friend(?), this person is not a true grownup.
3. Can this person cross the street without holding on to your hand? This may sound funny, but lots of friendships(?) are based on one person riding the other's energy, and then complaining about the direction or speed of the trip. If your friend(?) can't boil water, fill his/her own gas tank, or go to the store alone, this person is not grownup enough for you. You need to find someone who is self-sufficient and someone who welcomes a person of good company, like yourself.
4. Does this person still run away from home often? Most kids go through a stage where they threaten to run away from home, and some teenagers actually do it. This is difficult enough to deal with from a bona fide teenager. Don't put up with this for a minute from a suppose-to-be-adult friend. If this person goes through various periods of hot and cold, hide and seek, come here/go away, you know that this person is not a true grownup and is not able to be a true friend.

5. Does this person have to take long naps frequently (in front of the T.V., perhaps) even when they aren't really tired? One of the unmistakable marks of a true grownup is the ability to stay awake for one's life, or at least for long stretches of it at a time.

6. Does this person insist on fighting over toys and territory and who's boss of the game? Does this person cry or throw a fit when losing the hand or not getting his/her way? Does this person cheat when you're not looking? You need someone who is mature enough to play games fair and square, to be a gracious loser and winner. Even if your candidate for friendship learned how to be a team player as a child, this may not be enough. Grownup games require creative invention and negotiation about rules, roles, and rewards.

7. Can this person tell the difference between fantasy and reality? Is he/she brave enough to tell the truth to you and to him/her self? Can he/she be available to hear what is true for you? Is this person dedicated to discovering the truth in life situations or does he/she insist on playing "make-believe" and "let's pretend"? A rich fantasy life can be a valuable, creative resource but not when there is confusion or mislabeling of what is fantasy and what is reality. People who lie for convenience or say to others what they think others want to hear are not candidates for true friends and are not likely to become such any time soon.

8. Can this person identify and ask for what he/she needs? Can this person behave gracefully when you are unable to meet his/her requests? Infants and young children express their needs by crying, screaming, or looking miserable. Adults, then, use clever detective skills to find out what is really wrong and what might remedy the situation. If your friend is not able to identify and communicate his/her needs and accept disappointments gracefully a good deal of the time, he/she is not a true grownup.

In summary: Children, clients, patients, students, and even, in some instances, employees, may be people with potential. However, friends, spouses, and life partners must be capable of participating fully in equal partnerships. For you to experience this empowering opportunity, you must find people who are already true grownups. A good friend is someone who has *already arrived* at this place of response-ability. Good luck in using the above test to find friends who don't need you and who don't need you to need them! One of the most important ways to take care of yourself, to be selfcaring and selfhealing is to:

Give Yourself The Gift Of Grownup Friends.

Act Three

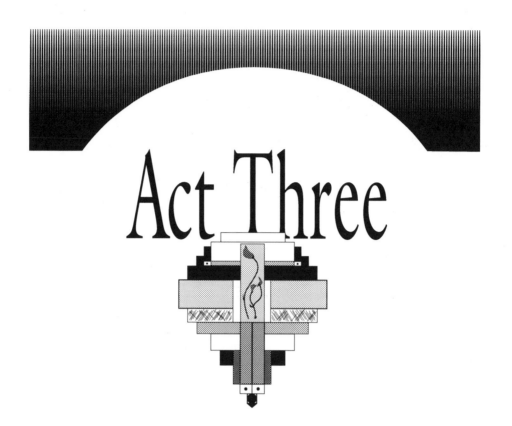

The Practice
and Rehearsal

The dancer is not separate from the dance, and all aspects
of the dancer are needed for the dance. Each of the next four chapters focuses
on one of the four dimensions of the self. Like weight, height,
and depth, our physical, mental, emotional and spiritual aspects together
describe a consistent whole. Like colors and shapes in a kaleidoscope,
turned slightly you highlight a particular pattern, turned again, the material
rearranges into a different pattern.

Part of our need to heal comes from our culture's division of these dimensions
into separate, unrelated domains presided over by isolated, often
warring experts. Physicians have claimed the physical; professors and scientists,
the mental; various mental health therapists, the emotional;
and ministers and priests, the spiritual. Like children playing "King of the Hill,"
each expert claims to be the most important one.

Even within ourselves the dimensions may seem to be competing for our
time and attention. The dance of selfhealing involves reclaiming
one's own authority over all of the dimensions of the self. Experts can be useful,
but they should work for us. The dance of selfcaring involves
a balanced relationship between all the dimensions. As we look at the dimensions
individually let's keep in mind their connections to one another.
*Selfcare isn't possible without slowing down **physically,** quieting the*
*mind **mentally**, allowing ourselves to experience and move*
*through feelings **emotionally,** and coming to realize **spiritually** that*
order will emerge out of what appears to be chaos.

Those move easiest
who have learned to dance.

Reclaiming and Reconditioning: The Physical

6

Like putty, we are either shaping ourselves or we are drooping; like clay,
we either keep ourselves moist and malleable or we are drying and hardening.
Deane Juhan, *Job's Body*[1]

"One, two, buckle my shoe. Three, four, touch the floor!" At one
time most of us were able to stay physically fit through the fun and
games of childhood pastimes. Jumping rope, running, riding bikes,
climbing trees, we developed strength and stamina, flexibility and the
ability to rest at the end of a hard day's play.

As we put away the things of our childhood many of us lost the
enjoyment of physical movement and the good feelings of experiencing our physical dimension. Staying physically fit (when we decide to
care about it at all) becomes serious work.

"One, two! Buckle those shoes! Three, four, touch the floor!" And
the beat goes on! Burn, Burn!" We do twenty of these and thirty of
those and repeat to ourselves, "No pain, no gain!" Pushing our bodies
a little farther, a little faster, we don't notice the muscle that says,
"enough"! And we forget to ask ourselves what is all this fitness for?

The recent body boom changed how we viewed our bodies and our
physical selves. At first we jumped right into exercise and fitness programs to stay healthy and young. It looked so easy on the video screen.
But then for many of us came the injuries. As it turns out, enthusiasm and
good intentions are not sufficient to insure a safe outcome.

Discouraged by overdoing, we then experienced periods of ignoring and denying our body's needs. We tell ourselves we "just aren't
athletic," "we don't have time," or "what's the use?"

What does fitness in the physical dimension mean for people
whose work involves caring for others? There are five aspects to
physical fitness: stamina, strength, flexibility, cardiovascular fitness,
and relaxation.[2] Stamina to marathon runners means being able to
withstand a long race. Stamina for peopleworkers is about how much
energy we have left over for our own lives after a long day at work.

Football players build strength to push back the line or to avoid being run over by a stronger team. Physical strength for caregivers may mean being able repeatedly to lift children or a sick elder without hurting oneself. Many caregivers like physical therapists, dentists, nurses, and beauticians need strength to survive being constantly on their feet. And it takes strength to hold a particular body posture for long periods of time, bending over a client or patient.

In sports like tennis and racket ball, flexibility enables players to respond quickly in changing directions. Some caregivers risk losing their flexibility as they sit for long periods of time listening to the needs of others. Doing paper work and talking on the phone can be more of the same rigid thing. Like everything in the physical dimension, using our flexibility is the only way to keep from losing it.

In sports, cardiovascular fitness means the body is able to respond when a sudden demand is made upon it and then to return quickly to a state of rest. Caregivers' hearts need these same abilities. Appreciating our needs in the physical dimension means recognizing our hearts and lungs require more opportunities for vigorous activity than most of our job and home tasks provide.

For the athlete, relaxation is an ease of movement which comes from an efficient use of the body. Peopleworkers need such efficiency as well. Along with the ability to let go of the stresses of caring work, we need the ability to rest for recovery and renewal. It is too late when exhaustion or pain signal our need for rest. Selfcare in the physical dimension means taking care of our needs before or as they arise. Like runners who are advised to keep drinking water during the race, by the time we experience thirst, the damage of dehydration has already begun.

HAZARDS OF IGNORING OUR PHYSICAL SELVES

Meeting our needs in an early stage requires paying close attention to our physical selves, but our training at all levels of schooling has sent us in the opposite direction. As first graders we lined up for the bathroom when school schedules dictated rather than listening and responding to our own inner signals. As junior high students we learned to gulp down lunch for more time on the playground. And should we exhibit too much physical movement in class, we were barred from the playground until we could learn to sit still.

High school and college found us losing sleep cramming for exams. Internships and training programs expected us to jump over the hurdles of long hours, little sleep, and an extended diet of junk food. As one physician participant in a workshop on selfcare expressed it, "As a student you really can't take care of yourself. Interns hold their breath and 'gun-it' through the training. Later, in practice, you try to find the shortcuts that make life bearable."

Think of the rituals in earning a professional degree or becoming licensed or certified for a particular field of work. Like fraternity pledges going through hazing, candidates pass the humiliation test and prove they can take what those in authority dish out. This sacrifice of our sensitivity is rendered on behalf of learning or science, selling or service, whatever at the time seems the noblest of causes.

What price do we pay for ignoring our own physical needs while living a caring-for-others lifestyle? We will look at three professional helpers and the particular physical difficulties they have encountered. We will see a caring lifestyle that consists of too little movement, one that contains too much, and a third that illustrates the danger in the way actions are performed.

The Case Of The Transfixed Therapist

Meet Rex, a 68 year old man who has been a psychotherapist for over 40 years. He sees 30 to 35 people each week, excepting the month of August and the two weeks he takes off each January. He came to one of Ilana Rubenfeld's workshops on selfcare for helping professionals complaining of stiffness and pain in his neck. A physician who x-rayed him told him that he had arthritis. Rex had concluded that there wasn't much he could do about his discomfort, but he volunteered to show the workshop leader and group how he sits when he is working with his clients.

A mock office was set up at the workshop, and Rex pretended to be working with a client. Ilana suggested he imagine a particular client, one that he considered especially difficult to work with. As Rex continued to imagine listening to his difficult client, his posture changed dramatically. When he was talking to the leader and the group, he was sitting upright with his spine elongated. As soon as he imagined his difficult client he sunk into his habitual listening pose.

"Freeze right where you are!" the leader directed. Like pushing the stop action frame on the video recorder, Rex became a still statue of his listening habit.

"Exaggerate that position," the leader added, hoping to further heighten his awareness of his listening habit. Rex's listening position meant that he was leaning forward, elbow on knee, sticking his neck out, chin on hand, somewhat reminiscent of the "thinker pose" of the famous statue. His eyes were focused straight ahead on the client. When asked to name this pose Rex exclaimed, "I'm Trance-fixed!"

He was correct. From his fixed position he could not move easily to the right or left. The strain of hour by hour, year by year, living in this position had cost him the loss of the rotational movement of his neck and spine. He felt stiffness and quite a bit of pain on occasion. He felt drained even before the end of each workday. Even the simple act of driving his car had become a dangerous activity since he could only look straight ahead.

The role that his mind was playing in all this became apparent when he was asked to experiment with listening to his clients from different positions. He explored postures that were less strenuous for him, sitting back in his chair which meant moving further away from the client. When a position felt physically comfortable for him, he worried about giving the wrong message to his clients.

> "I feel that they will think I am not listening to them, that I don't care about them or their problems," Rex said.

The leader invited Rex to experiment with listening to people from these more comfortable positions and postures as he interacted with people at the workshop. Since workshop participants weren't paying for his time like clients, Rex was able to experiment with the more comfortable listening postures and get reactions from others as to how he came across.

After some experimentation, Rex began to loosen his fixed notions about how to be with others as a helping person. As he allowed more flexibility in his physical positions, he relaxed emotionally and mentally. This allowed more aspects of himself to show through to his colleagues at the workshop. The real test came, of course, when he was back home listening to his clients.[3]

THE IMPORTANCE OF POSTURE

Improper posture is a most significant energy drainer in our daily lives. As we carry out the tasks of work and home life, the answer isn't just to "sit up straight" or "put your shoulders back" as most of us have been advised to do as children. Posture isn't a position. Posture is a relationship between all parts of our bodies as we engage in the movements of living. As Rex clearly demonstrated, our posture reflects our attitude about ourselves and others and our beliefs about what it takes to achieve what we are trying to accomplish.

Whatever techniques we have developed to accomplish actions such as sitting in a chair, walking, swinging a golf club, or brushing our teeth, we have achieved some level of proficiency. After years of practice we are unaware of what we are doing to accomplish these tasks, but, whatever it is, it feels natural and necessary. Many of these techniques, like Rex's listening posture, may be costing us our energy and good health in the long run.

Around the turn of the century, the Shakespearean actor F. M. Alexander discovered this truth when he developed laryngitis frequently as he practiced his acting craft. Since this was before the invention of public address systems, he might have just considered this illness an occupational hazard. Instead, he reasoned that there might be something in the way he was using his physical self which created the problems with his voice. Observing himself with mirrors from many angles (video cameras hadn't been invented yet), he became aware of what he was doing with his head and neck as he performed his dramatic work. He identified what he came to call his "misuse of self" in posture and movement which inhibited his voice and created his frequent bouts with laryngitis.

Alexander also found that changing these unproductive habits was not as easy as it looked. He eventually developed the Alexander Method, a system of psychophysical education which helps people learn to treat themselves more gently as they perform daily tasks.[3]

PRACTICING A NEW POSTURE

Remember, healthy posture is not a position but a relationship between parts which allows for ease of movement and a lack of strain. Try the following activity to get an understanding of the importance of Alexander's discovery.

1) Go through the motions of what you usually do at work in slow motion.
2) At some point in the process, freeze.
3) Notice the fine detail of the position of your head and neck in space. (Is your chin jutting forward? Is your forehead reaching out beyond your chest?) The desired movement is for your head to move subtly back and up, so let's practice by starting with exaggerating the opposite.
4) Place one palm across your forehead and the other on the back of your neck. Move your chin forward and notice how your neck is shortened.
5) Move your forehead back and allow your chin to drop and the back of your neck to lengthen.
6) Grasp several hairs from the crown of your head and gently guide your head in an upwardly direction, lengthening the spine as you go.

7) Now perform your work tasks from this new posture and experience the lightness and ease of movement.
8) Notice which old habits cause you to lose this new posture.
9) To reclaim your new posture repeat steps 4 through 6.

THE IMPORTANCE OF MODERATION

Besides posture and the problem of too little movement, a caring lifestyle can involve too much movement. Let's meet another caregiver who illustrates that type of problem .

REVEREND PERPETUAL MOTION

No disrespect intended. People call her Reverend Perpetual Motion — to her face! Dr. Karen Rutledge, the hospital chaplain is the closest thing to a perpetual motion machine you'll ever see. She's up the stairs two at a time and down in a flash when her pager sounds its beep. Karen is 48, but you'd never know it. Her energy seems boundless. She appears to be working every shift, often coming back to the hospital on weekends and evenings. She grabs a hamburger on the run, and nobody can figure out when she sleeps.

"My job is supporting parents and staff through the difficult times in the treatment (and sometimes death) of the children who are our patients," Karen said. "It's a perfect job for me, though I didn't have this situation in mind when I went to the seminary. I thought at the time I would have my own church. But this assignment feels like real pastoral care. It brings together all my interests and skills from my years as a teacher, mother, and community volunteer. The only shadow on the horizon is that I have just discovered I have a health problem. When I was having trouble getting over the flu I went to the doctor, and he tells me I have had a mild heart attack. There is heart trouble in my family, but I didn't experience any warning signs. In the back of my mind, I knew I wasn't eating right or getting enough sleep, but I thought the good feelings I had from my job would carry me through."

ATTENDING TO OUR PHYSICAL SELVES

Our bodies cannot stay healthy when we tend to others and forget to attend to ourselves. As Julian Silverman suggests in his book, *Health Care and Consciousness*,[4] our habit of living in our heads doesn't allow us to be healthy. Our bodies can not stay in balance without the energy that some degree of attention provides. As soon as we pay attention to our bodies we begin to make a difference. This information which only the body can give helps us to know what we need, what to do next, and how to alter our course.

Because of our special sensitivity to others, we caregivers have to overcome a tendency to lose track of ourselves and our own needs while relating to others. Sometimes it would be quite accurate for us to hang a sign on our chests, the kind shopkeepers hang on their doors: "GONE FISHING!" or "NOBODY HOME!" or a special one for mothers, "BE BACK IN 20 YEARS!"

A physical illness is often the signal that gets our attention, and we start to get the message "we aren't invincible."

Karen's selfhealing journey began when the doctor told her she had a heart condition. Her selfcaring journey began when she stopped thinking of herself as a sprinter and began regarding herself as a long distance runner.

Karen began systematically to change her lifestyle. Her first decision was to treat herself to a weekly therapeutic massage. Though this seemed self indulgent to her at first, she soon realized that through the skilled touch of the body worker she was developing a consciousness about her body. As Deane Juhan described it,

Touching hands are not like pharmaceuticals or scalpels. They are like flashlights in a darkened room. The medicine they administer is self-awareness.[5]

Growing out of Karen's emerging self awareness of her body came a commitment to focus on what, how, and when she was eating. She joined forces with a nutritionist, and together they systematically looked at how her body was digesting and assimilating what she was eating. She learned that nourishment isn't just whether you can digest that hamburger, but it is about what happens to the cells. Karen described her reactions to the process this way:

"At first hearing, I seldom welcomed any suggestions made to me to alter my eating habits. Intellectually, I had dozens of excuses why the suggestion was too much trouble or wouldn't work. Emotionally, I felt threatened that I would be losing something important or trading something enjoyable for something distasteful. I achieved the best results through being willing to try a small change for a short period of time. As each small change produced a benefit in my system, I got the courage to try another."

● ●

DEVELOPING A HEALTHY RELATIONSHIP WITH FOOD

Here are some suggestions for moving towards a selfcaring lifestyle as far as food and physical nourishment are concerned. Consider, as some clients have done, copying these suggestions and fastening them on your refrigerator door.

1. Don't make dramatic or drastic changes in your diet as this is stress-producing. Slow and steady adjustments are more likely to be maintained. Should you develop an adverse reaction to some dietary change, it's easier to identify the cause of the difficulty if alterations are introduced one at a time.

2. If your habit is to use food as your drug of choice to stuff unpleasant feelings or create positive ones, work with a therapist to learn healthy ways to handle feelings.

3. Keep your food and dietary planning simple or you won't be able to stick with it. Shop for and prepare foods on the weekends so you can eat healthfully during your work week.

4. If your plan is to lose weight or let go of your addictive foods, join a group such as Overeaters Anonymous for support.

5. Stay skeptical of "quick fixes" in the nutritional area as well as in other areas of your life.

6. When the time seems right, consider working with a nutritionist or a doctor who specializes in preventive medicine.

7. Begin substituting intermediate foods for unhealthy ones, (cookies sweetened with fruit juice replacing cookies with sugar, decaf coffee or herb teas replacing caffeinated drinks).

8. Make breakfast your biggest meal (include protein) and supper your lightest (soup and salad). This helps you get a good night's sleep.

9. Help your elimination system by taking two glasses of water with lemon juice upon rising, followed by moderate exercise such as walking. This morning ritual flushes out toxins and gets the system ready for the day.

10. Develop other ways to comfort or nurture yourself physically besides using food. Consider luxurious hot baths, massages, and the gift of some quiet time.

11. Include exercise in your selfcaring nutritional plan since exercise plays an important part in helping your body use what you are feeding it.

12. Alter grandma's recipes in the direction of lower fat and less sugar so you and your family can still enjoy them.

13. Try out these healthy variations of old recipes when you bring food to the office for parties or coffee breaks. This way the culture of the office can become supportive of eating in a selfcaring way.

14. Occasionally disobey the rules of whatever plan you design so that you don't become rigid, resentful, or arrogant.

15. Begin or revive a ritual of expressing gratitude for the gift of good food before and after meals, even when eating alone. This can be as simple as a moment of attentive silence or as elaborate as your traditions recommend.

The Importance Of Balance

Our third professional helper illustrates what happens when you not only do too much, but it is done too intensely and without the balance provided by other types of experiences. Marie's life had become all work. In addition to being a professional helper, she has been a professional student working part-time to finish her degree in psychology.

Marie The Magnificent

"I'm nearly 30 years old and this is my eighth year of going to school for this degree. After I finish this next round of tests I still have a dissertation to write and an internship to go through," Marie told me on her first visit to my office.

"I believe that stressful times can be opportunities for growth," Marie said, "but I am losing confidence that I can grow from these next few months of exams and faculty reviews."

Marie was having trouble sleeping. She was experiencing numbness in her fingers and tension headaches. She felt guilty whenever she took time from her studies. Having little time with her husband caused trouble in her marriage. Marie and I discussed her approach to achieving her educational goals. Her success was impressive—straight A grades, outstanding student awards, truly a magnificent record. Overdoing had been her strategy. Doing "her best " meant studying "every waking moment," and this had worked for many years. But now, when the stakes were higher than ever, she was worn out. Angry at the price she had been paying, she felt unsure of herself and panicked at the idea of letting people down. And of course, she didn't want to destroy that superwoman image she had so carefully constructed through the years.

Marie's story hasn't ended yet. I suggested ways to become more selfcaring. I introduced her to some ways to let up on herself, and ways to become aware of her physical self. She rejected any suggestion that she relax her lofty standards. She chose to continue pushing herself even harder to "get it over with."

"I'll start taking care of myself after I get my degree," she told me. Having been there myself and having observed many social work students make the same decision, I knew that, after graduation, there would be a price to pay. Given the symptoms she was already experiencing, I expressed my hope that she not injure herself irreversibly in this process of achieving near perfection. I let the matter drop in the interest of my own selfcare. I told her I would be available to work with her on her recovery when she felt ready to do so.

RECLAIMING OUR PHYSICAL SELVES

Overdoing teaches many of us the necessity of taking care of ourselves. Bodies neglected for too long show disastrous results and suggest the necessity of reclaiming our bodies and learning to love them. Many people are dissatisfied with their bodies, wanting to be taller or thinner, or they disrespect its limitations. Maybe it's your thighs or chest that don't meet your expectations! The list is potentially endless, and the constant struggle puts us at odds with vital parts of ourselves. It is important to remember that our bodies are not only vehicles to transport brains. Our bodies are a significant aspect of who we are, and appreciating, respecting, and loving our physical selves is a significant part of appreciating and loving ourselves. We have heard the stories of three caregivers and their experiences with the physical effects resulting from their work stress. For some additional help with this dimension, let's consult with the Soma Twins. Remember — she is sensory, he is motor — so they should have much to teach us about taking care of our physical selves.

The Soma Twins On The Stress Systems

I asked the twins to explain what it is that happens physically when people who care for others burn out. Touchy responsed, "The importance of posture and how our mental attitude affects it was illustrated by Rex, the transfixed therapist. He was caught in the possum response — inactivity to the point of rigid stillness. This reaction is self protection for a possum as he "plays dead" to fool his enemies, but it doesn't work for people. The stress of staying in one place habitually takes its toll in loss of flexibility, range of movement, and the sensitivity to be in touch with your own needs."

Feelie added, "All the different stress responses are costly over the long haul. Overdoing, as Karen and Marie described, is costly when continued over extended periods of time. When the 'fight or flight' response of the sympathetic nervous system (arousal) goes on for too long, it depletes the body's resources and puts strain on major organs like the heart, liver, and lungs. If the parasympathetic nervous system (inhibition) is active for too long, the immune system becomes depressed, leading to susceptibility to a wide range of diseases from mental depression to cancer.[6] Sometimes people feel drained and used up, yet like Marie they are unable to relax and replenish themselves. Others turn off, toughen up, and hold on to their tension. Like Rex, they can't express themselves, and they won't allow themselves to receive from others. All of this places tremendous stress on the body."

Touchy described a remedy. "Two systems of the nervous system (sympathetic and parasympathetic) need to be in balance in order for people to experience health and well being. Instead of thinking of relaxation as regulated by an on/off switch, picture a rheostat knob which allows you to brighten and dim the lights with a great deal of variety. If doing (action) and non-doing (relaxation) are operated by a rheostat knob, then each combination creates a particular body/mind state. For each task, activity, and skill there is an optimum body/mind state, and the possibilities for unique and creative combinations are infinite."

Feelie adds: "When a person is able to relax (and there are different levels of this in the body), anything extraneous is deleted. When movement becomes a dance, only what is necessary to the movement is activated and only to the appropriate level."

Touchy concluded, "From the point of view of the stress systems, all elements of fitness rely on relaxation; the ability to release excess tension and inhibit unnecessary activity."

"Dancers and master athletes perfect their technique by developing the ability to sense small changes in balance, position in space, and breathing," said Feelie. "This kind of sensitivity isn't possible when there is excess tension or a bracing within the body. Caring people are already sensitive to others so becoming selfcaring means heightening our sensitivity to ourselves as well."

MOVEMENTS FOR MENDING

As any young child will tell you, being made to sit still is a punishment. Our need for movement is as powerful as our need for food and rest. Fortunately, children's games provide rich opportunities for different kinds of movement. Most kids wouldn't consider giving up moving unless, while playing "Hide and Seek", the seeker comes too close to your hideout. Then you flatten down, suspend all movement including breathing, and hope that you have escaped discovery. Once discovered, it just means you will be **IT** in the next round of play.

Like the children's game of "statues," changing the way we move and the position of our bodies in space provides us with an interesting escape from habitual ways of being in the world. Since everything is connected, moving our bodies means that we are freeing our minds as well. You are invited to experiment with the Movements For Mending in Appendix B. Intersperse these activities into your daily schedule as a way to develop further your ability to relax, your flexibility, and your strength. And notice any difference this movement makes in your stamina at the end of the day. As you heighten sensitivity to your own body, what is needed for balance becomes obvious, and balance is the essence of selfcaring.

PHYSICAL ACTIVITIES AND SELFCARING

As an aid to selecting other physical activity, consider the guide in Appendix A The Guide To Selecting Physical Activity is a series of questions, the answers to which may assist you in evaluating any physical activities from the perspective of their contribution to selfcaring and selfhealing.

If your chosen activity doesn't pass this test, ask yourself if it is the way you are doing the activity. You may need to lighten up in your approach. (Remember the book,"Inner Tennis"?) Ask yourself, what kind of an inner dance instructor or coach do I have? You may need to contact or build one that is more congruent with your need for selfcaring and selfhealing.

Who Is Your Inner Instructor?

How we treat ourselves in our inner world has been strongly affected by the teachers and coaches of our youth. You may be having trouble maintaining your sensitivity and staying in a selfcaring attitude towards yourself due to the type of instructors you actually experienced. You may have met the dance instructor, Madam Haughty Hanna. Not having taken care of herself as she aged, she now uses a cane which she pounds continuously on the floor.

She doesn't mind using the cane to pound her students should they dare to make a mistake. Her special enjoyment is teaching by humiliation, ridiculing her students' physical characteristics, and attacking their personalities if they, even momentarily, seem to feel good about themselves.

Another damaging type of instructor or coach is one I call Hurly-Burly Harold. He and the others of his ilk are graduates of the *Kick Butt School of Instruction* and should be avoided at all costs. This cigar smoking, potbellied weasel tells his team members that they played such a lousy first half they can't possibly win. He adds insults to his injury by making remarks about how they played like "girls, queers, and pansies!" (It is not clear why this particular flower is picked out for insult, but it seems to add fuel to his fire.)

Both of these instructors hope that the students' hatred of the one who mistreated them will motivate them to do the near impossible and prove their instructors wrong. When the athletes do win, or the dancers perform well, comments are made such as "How come it took so long?" Students are also reminded that this just proves they could have performed well all along.

Another version of this type is the gym teacher who teaches his students how to hate physical activity and their own bodies as well. Punishment for misbehavior becomes laps around the gym, or better yet, around the school grounds. That way the kids can get sick from exposure to inclement weather and peers can share their humiliation as well.

An Inner Instructor Of Another Kind

In spite of the large number of Madam Haughty Hannas and Hurly Burly Harolds, another type of instructor has been emerging on the scene in recent years. This teacher sees her job as the development of the inner dancer or athlete. Her philosophy is not that winning is everything, but rather that, everything that happens is a win. She instructs her students to repeat the following affirmation before each practice and each game or performance.

> **I am as important as any one or all of my projects, goals, and accomplishments—past, present, and future. I will allow myself to be fully present to the task at hand, realizing that, whatever happens, I will learn from it.**

This instructor, Ivy the Instiller, seeks to develop in her students a sense of attention and focus, an attitude of discovery, an ability to make mistakes and learn from them, the ability to allow confusion and sometimes not to know the answers. Most of all, Ivy insists her students learn how to play.

You might want to develop your own Inner Ivy. She's the kind of person who, when all of the members of the gymnastic team fell off the high bars during an important meet, fastened the following note to the dressing room door:

Hey, Team!
Falling is not a giant zap from the gods
meant to embarrass, humiliate, and hurt you, but
falling is one of the things that happens
in the process of "going for it,"
as you move too close to your growing edge.
It is a sign that you have made an error
and you need to;

BREATHE........as in keep breathing.
LAUGH..........as in keep releasing.
GET UP.........as in keep moving.
LAUGH..........as in keep enjoying.

and get back on the horse,
ring, barre, or floor!

SMILE......... as you uncover, discover,
recover, the lessons of each particular fall.

Summary

In living a selfcaring lifestyle we are affected by habits of the past, beliefs we have about ourselves and about how others view us, and the feelings and attitudes we bring to the helping situation. The dance of selfcaring in the physical dimension involves . . .

Movement

affecting *posture* and *attitude*

which affects *breathing*

which affects *energy*

resulting in becoming DRAINED or ENERGIZED.

Those who dance are thought mad
by those who hear not the music.

Recalling and Revisioning: The Mental

7

The mind is the source of liberation as well as of bondage.
The Upanishads

Becoming selfcaring frequently involves selfhealing our past. In order to move forward in our lives we may need to recall significant memories and reframe them as positive resources for our present and future. This is the crux of what most mental health therapy is about, but often the memories are not easily accessible while in a discussion format. Memories of past traumas remain locked in our bodies while we struggle to reason our way to health. In order to make sense of the information gleaned from various health care experts, selfhealing requires that we reconnect our bodies with our minds and learn various ways of working with our own mental dimension.

FORGOTTEN MEMORIES AND SELFHEALING

Our way of being in the world (the amount of tension we carry, what we expect from ourselves) is a natural response to events in our early life. Sometimes in order to change unhealthy habits, we need to learn new ones and come to some understanding about the situations that stimulated our early responses. All this can seem overwhelmingly complicated unless we discover a way to make the connection between then and now and learn a way to think differently about the past.

THE CASE OF THE LOST CHILD WITHIN

Meet Alice, a teacher of children in special education, who had a lot to learn from her own special child within.

When Alice and I met she had already been to many doctors and experienced various types of physical therapies. She had tried medication, biofeedback, and just about anything else anyone suggested. Her problem, which had been going on for two years by that time, was a chronic pain in her right shoulder. Alice was referred to me by one of my former students who knew I did a kind of therapy which involved mental, emotional, and spiritual aspects of physical problems. On the intake sheet Alice had written, "You are my last hope."

I declined to occupy such a position of power over her future. I told her honestly that I did not know if I could help her but I was willing, if she was, to form a partnership to see what we could do together about the situation. I explained the work I would be doing with her, the Rubenfeld Synergy Method. We would begin by helping her to develop a fine-tuned awareness of her body. I would use gentle touch to focus and highlight her awareness. I would assist her to let go of extra habitual tension she might be carrying. If that tension were connected to any events in her life, past or present, we would deal with that aspect as well.

Slowly but steadily Alice and I discovered more about her physical self. Not surprisingly her upper body, particularly her shoulders, were in a state of hypertension and unable to let go and relax. Her lower body (pelvis and legs) seemed to be too loose and lacking the strength to really support her.

Mentally Alice never stopped for a minute. She corrected students' papers in the waiting room before her sessions with me. She made lists and outlines and planned what she was cooking for dinner. We discovered that the only time she took time out to relax was when her shoulder pain became severe. Then, in spite of her strong sense of duty, she delegated responsibility for dinner to her husband and children. Then, in pain, she allowed herself to sit in a recliner in her bedroom with a heating pad on her shoulder.

"One good thing this shoulder pain does for you is to give you some time to yourself to rest and recuperate," I said. "Do you think you could take care of yourself like that *without* your shoulder hurting?"

After a great deal of effort trying to imagine the situation I was proposing, Alice answered. "Maybe I could, but it would sure be a whole lot harder."

As months went by in our work together, Alice made small changes in the way she treated herself. She became more selfcaring, allowing others to take over family chores, even when she wasn't in pain. This meant giving up the perfectionist way she *thought* things should be done. One day as I was working with her on releasing her shoulder she said, "It feels like there is a little fist inside that shoulder blade."

I asked her to make a fist with her hand and she noted that when she did that, the "little fist" inside her shoulder seemed to ease a bit. When Alice returned the following week, she reported a memory she had had while lying in bed.

"I don't know if this has anything to do with anything, but I remembered that, as a child, I always pulled the covers up to my chin, and I'd sleep with my hands clutching the blanket." As she demonstrated the sleeping position, we both noted the raised position of her shoulders. This position was quite similar to the bracing posture she walked around in habitually when we first met.

In the weeks that followed, the quality of our work together become more playful. Alice allowed herself to remember games and toys that she had loved as a child. It was during one of those playful, relaxing sessions that she suddenly looked up at me and said, matter of factly, "When I was growing up, my parents were both alcoholics. Could that have anything to do with all of this?"

As we continued our discussion, Alice remembered why she slept in that clutched position. She would go to bed, night after night, to the sound of her parents fighting. After she fell asleep, she would be awakened by their loud, aggressive voices.

Remembering the situation which created the posture enabled her to heal. Releasing her chronically tight shoulders meant she reexperienced the feelings of fear and anger. Letting go of her anger and fear allowed her to further let go of the tension in her shoulders.

ELEMENTS OF SELFCARING

Many elements of selfcaring and selfhealing are illustrated in Alice's story. She had "forgotten" her early childhood experiences, both pleasant as well as unpleasant. This left her in a state of constant physical and mental vigilance. Overdoing in her caretaking role, she had forgotten how to *play* or receive *support* from others. As she became more selfcaring she was able to *rest* without the excuse of pain. She was able to recall her past, reconnect with her inner child, and reframe her view of how she needed to be in the world now, as an adult. After she stopped bracing and continually getting ready for some unknown danger, she regained the ability to *rest*, receive *nourishment*, and enjoy *pleasure, play,* and *laughter*.

USING OUR MINDS

Researchers are just beginning to understand the way that memories, experience, and learning are stored and retrieved in the body/mind. In order to develop confidence in the ability of one's mind to act on one's own behalf (to help take care of oneself), some understanding is needed of the complexity of such everyday experiences as remembering and forgetting.

According to Ernest Rossi, who reviewed hundreds of research articles on how the brain communicates with the body, all learning takes place in a particular body/mind state.[1] Most often, these states are not immediately accessible to what we call our "conscious mind". Sometimes these different states can be so separated from each other that they create separate personalities (as in the movie "The Three Faces of Eve").

THE SOMA TWINS AND THE STRESS RESPONSE

Let's call on the Soma Twins to help us understand the way we can work with our mental dimension for selfhealing and selfcaring.

Touchy began. "It shouldn't be too surprising that we lose some of our great ideas when you realize there are 2 times one hundred million possible mental states in each person's brain."

Feelie added," One of the major difficulties for people in understanding and working with the mental dimension is the notion that all prior learnings are stored somewhere in their head. Most people don't realize what Karl Pribram, the brain researcher has discovered. Mental images and content are not stored in little files in the brain but constructed each time they are accessed."

"And here's where we come in," Touchy said. "This reconstruction involves not only the brain but sensory and motor aspects of the body as well. We work closely with the hypothalamus, a special tissue about the size of a pea at the base of the forebrain."

Feelie joined in. "The hypothalamus receives the electrical impulses Touchy and I are sending from all parts of the nervous system. It integrates this information with the cognitive part of the mind (cerebral cortex) and then releases hormones to regulate a particular tissue of the body. Hormones are the messenger molecules which travel from the brain via the endocrine system (including the pituitary), altering the state of the body."

"Let's give a practical example," said Touchy. "Imagine you are on an airplane, reading, and the plane is in flight. You have a sensation of flutter in your stomach. You think 'Oops, this airplane just hit an air pocket.' Your hypothalamus sends a messenger molecule to the stomach which first perceived the imbalance. This turns *off* the butterflies and other flutters of the body's alarm system."

"On the other hand," Touchy continued, "if the hypothalamus receives the following message from the mind: 'THIS IS IT ! —Doomsday!...The end of the world!' The messenger molecules traveling from your brain via the endocrine system (including the pituitary) will then alter the body state. The body responds with : *'Turn on stress response'* "

Feelie explained, "So, the limbic-hypothalamic system of the brain is the central switching station. By receiving energy from one system (autonomic nerve, endocrine, or immune) and integrating it with mental processes (sensory, perceptual, emotional, and cognitive), this communication system plays an important part, not only in memory, but in learning, stress reduction, and healing."

I told the twins, "There are two things that stand out for me in what you are saying. In our culture we forget that there are other kinds of thought forms in the mind besides conscious analytical thought and the arrangement of logical sequences. The second part of this is that the body is capable of many kinds of thought forms connected to the five senses. Intelligence and memory are functioning even in the tiniest cell."

Feelie agreed, "The other kinds of thought forms include feeling states, sensory memories, focused imaginings, and kinetic memories. In fact, in order for these other forms to operate, we need to stop analyzing and commanding from the front brain."

"Anyone who has survived an important exam during schooling or professional training can attest to the fact that a certain level of relaxation and a lessening of anxiety is necessary in order to make connections with what we know," said Touchy.

"The converse is also true, extreme anxiety and trauma can cause people to become amnesic about an event or period of their life. In fact, in order to recall a memory, it is often necessary to reenter or recreate the body/mind state which existed at the time of the initial learning or event," Feelie concluded.

Muscle Memory

After my discussion with the twins, I remembered something dancers and athletes call "muscle memory." I guess now it more accurately should be called "whole body memory." Here the person doesn't *think* about a tennis stroke or series of dance steps but goes back through the motions and the body remembers. The athletic coach says, "Practice the stroke the way I taught you until it gets in your body and you don't have to think about it."

As a choreographer's assistant, I had some unusual experiences with the part my body played in remembering. Choreographers create dances. They try the steps and patterns out on assistants who then teach the dance to other dancers. Choreographers seldom remember their own dances, especially if a lot of time has elapsed since they created them. After a dance has been performed many times and then retired from the repertoire, I would be called upon to help reconstruct it. Even though I had performed the dance hundreds of times, I could recall very little of it consciously. But when the music was played and I began dancing the movements, my body began remembering one phrase after another. This method would only carry me so far, and then I would draw a blank. I'd back up both the music and myself and "take it from the top," as they say in the theater. With each run through, my body would remember additional phrases until a twenty minute piece would finally be reconstructed. One particularly interesting thing about this method of recall was that my body would remember the first version of the dance, not subsequent revisions or additions.

• •

Test Your Muscle Memory

1) Select an activity — a dance, game, or sport that you used to engage in but have not experienced for many years. It could be riding a bicycle or scooter, playing hop scotch, or dancing a polka. How about kick the can? or marbles? How long has it been since you climbed a tree?

2) In order not to alert your stress response, stay in a place of pleasure, play, and laughter. The outcome of this experiment has no earth shaking consequences— just the opportunity to explore your own "muscle memory" and learn to trust it.

3) As you perform the activity, take notice of whether you simultaneously remember people or other aspects of the situations where you engaged in the activity years ago. If

so, consider this a bonus and reward for your willingness to put aside your adult "pride" and "dignity" in order to experience the clear sensory memories of *doing.*

MISUSE OF THE MIND

Several years ago, as my colleagues and I moved into new office space, we found a poster left behind by the former tenants. Its title was: "Seven Ways To Stagnate." We laughed at the familiarity of the items. There was nothing new on the list. We had heard all those reasons before:

"It won't work."

"It costs too much money."

"We tried that last year."

"It will take too long."

"Nobody will come (or buy or participate)."

"It will take too much work and it's a dumb idea, anyhow."

"*They* won't like it!"

In working with clients, I am often reminded of this poster and its reference to misuse of the reasoning mind. Cynthia was a nurse who had developed elaborate ways to stop herself from doing anything that was creative. And most of all, she stopped herself from looking forward to anything with enjoyment.

"Whenever I start to feel good about something, like the conference I am organizing for new nursing graduates, I start scaring myself by saying 'what if....?' Then I come up with all the possible catastrophes I can imagine. I find myself picturing the most preposterous circumstances like, 'what if the lady who is bringing the refreshments has her baby two months early and isn't able to bring them?' "

"I had another client once who played what he called the "Devil's Advocate game," I told Cynthia. "He'd think about doing something: taking a class, looking for another job, or asking a woman for a date. Then he would construct all the reasons why he shouldn't do any of those things. He was such an expert Devil's Advocate that he seldom ever attempted to do any of the things he initially thought of doing."

AFFIRMING THE AFFIRMATIVE

In working with the mind, rather than concentrating on the glass being half empty, we need to elaborate on the picture of what a full glass would look like. Rather than living in fear that we might lose its contents, the work is to imagine how it might be if it were overflowing.

I asked Cynthia to describe the conference she was preparing to present from the point of view of the best possible outcome. She stated, "I would like to enjoy the preparation I am going through, and look forward to a positive and successful outcome."

I introduced her to the idea of rehearsing for how she wanted things to turn out. Together, we created an affirmation, a statement which encompassed her desires:

> **"I am preparing for the conference and enjoying the process of preparation.'"**

The first reaction she had to what seemed a kind of Pollyanna thinking was, "What if I can't get everything done that needs doing?"

I asked her, "Are you the only person working on this project?"

"There are other people," Cynthia said, "but I have trouble trusting others to do what they say they will do." We added a second affirmation to the first:

> **"I am acting with others to insure a successful conference, and I am developing confidence in myself and others to successfully carry out our responsibilities."**

• •

Actions For Affirming[2]

1) Select something that you want to accomplish and state it in the positive, as though it were already occurring. Example:

> **"I am enjoying studying for my exam. I am successfully taking the exam from a place of comfort and confidence."**

2) Listen carefully for any objections to be raised from your sensory awareness. You might experience a feeling of uncomfortableness or hear a voice of objection, "What about.........." (Remember the seven ways to stagnate.)

3) Resolve that objection by using the selfcaring skills:

SORTING AND SEPARATING - "That was true when I was a child, but now, I am a grown person".

LETTING GO - Imagine the objections becoming surrounded by a cloud and floating up, up and away.

Using PARTNERSHIP POWER - "Together, I and my friend, (therapist, Higher Power, spirit guide) can do this."

STEPPING BACK - Allow yourself a panoramic perspective. See how things look from a satellite in outer space. How will the situation look 10 years from now?

EXERCISING CHOICE - Give yourself permission to believe in the possibility of a positive outcome. As Bernie Seigel suggests, "When faced with uncertainty, there's nothing wrong with hope."

THE EVERYDAY TRANCE

Selfcaring and selfhealing require that the logical left brain quiet itself so that we may experience who we truly are and what life is all about. One way that this occurs is in the everyday trance, which is a period of relaxation when the analytic mind is not in control. Nothing like the nightclub entertainer swinging his watch chain, trance states occur spontaneously every day. You drive your car on automatic pilot (a trance state) while thinking of what's for supper. You daydream (a trance state) during a pause in the proceedings at work. You suddenly notice that you have been singing to yourself for sometime (auditory hallucination) or you experience a *trance*-forming feeling of calm as you walk softly on new snow or stand silently overlooking a breathtaking view of the valley below. When we don't have the time or the ability to relax in these ways, we begin to experience stress from the inside, and we become unable to move forward in living our lives creatively.

FROM CRITICAL TO CREATIVE

"I have been so critical of my husband lately, I really feel guilty," Doris told me on our first visit in six or seven years. "You were really helpful to me when I was considering marrying Steve, so I thought of you when I had a particularly bad week.

I've thought my problem was hormones or maybe allergies, but checking those out hasn't given me any real answers."

I encouraged Doris to continue to follow the recommendations of her other doctors, but I felt there were some things we could do together that might uncover what this hypercritical attitude was all about. Consciously, Doris knew that she was treating her husband like her father had treated her.

"I always hated that behavior, and I don't want to become like my father at this stage of my life," Dois said.

Doris had taken leave from her job as a manager to complete a manuscript about working with handicapped children. She had been inspired to do this during a meditation retreat several years ago but she was having trouble finishing the book. "Do you think your critical attitude has anything to do with the scary thing you have done in taking your leave?" I asked.

"Well, I don't feel very good about myself," Doris admitted, "since I'm not making the progress I intended to make by now. I have all kinds of plans and good ideas as I'm getting ready for bed, but the next morning is a different story. I keep getting distracted by errands I need to run or laundry that hasn't been done. This working at home isn't as easy as it looks."

As Doris began to deal with her feelings about herself, she recognized her disappointment in not living up to her own expectations. Then she discovered how critical and mean she was to herself. "I guess it's no wonder I'm critical of my husband sometimes," she said.

Since one of her main difficulties was taking action when she needed and wanted to accomplish something, I suggested she participate in a movement group I was leading on a weekly basis. (Through movement games and activities this group assists members in getting out of their critical minds and into a responsive body consciousness.) Doris was reticent at first, saying she didn't have a sense of rhythm, she always felt uncomfortable about her body, and she never could think of anything to do that was original. (More ways to stagnate!)

Changing Doris's mind about herself began as soon as she learned how to allow herself to go into a state of relaxation or trance at the beginning of the group. At first she reported "falling asleep," but eventually she began to experience images as in a waking dream. The group helped her act out the image of herself standing in her kitchen, confused over what to do next, over-reasoning to the point of paralysis.

Some members took the roles of her resistances, physically holding her back from the forward movement she was trying to accomplish. Other members shouted, "Come on, Doris, you can do it! Don't let them get you down! We're rooting for you!"

"It sounds crazy," Doris said, "but in the middle of that activity in the movement group I realized that I'm afraid to act in any direction because I'll make a mistake. I'll be criticized. And if nobody else criticizes, the 'critical father' inside me will take over and do me in."

"Much of what you learned about yourself under the critical eyes of your father is not true," I told Doris. "I see you learning in the group that you do have rhythm and you can create original actions as long as you don't *think* too hard about it."

Therapeutic Trance

As Doris discovered, information, in trance states, may be generated or recalled with ease. Healing occurs when the re-creation of the memory can be done with some significant difference from the original event. Positive feelings are present as well as negative ones. Rather than experiencing the isolation of the original negative situation, you are in the presence of at least one other person, or you are working with a tool for transforming the situation to produce a different outcome. Doris achieved a breakthrough by re-enacting a difficult situation in the movement group. You can try this method of bypassing your critical self by following the directions in *Movements For Mending* in Appendix. Other ways to access your creative self are to use drawing or some other art techniques which access the imagery side of the brain. (See movement IX in appendix B.)

The Power Of An Image

According to Jeanne Achterberg[3], a powerful source of our creativity is the mind's ability to image. Imagery, more than just creating pictures, is the thought process that invokes and uses the senses.[3] Whether seeing or smelling, hearing or tasting, touching, sensing movement and position in space, these are all ways that the body / mind communicates with itself. In this two-way street, our bodies are affected by images that we hold, and the wisdom of our bodies can generate images. We can construct new images or call to mind images we need to remember for our healing.

Healing A Self Image

Meet Peggy, a social work administrator who, at age 40,

finally began learning what it meant to take care of herself. On a disability leave from her job at the state school for the retarded when I first met her, Peggy had a long history of doing a good job for her clients and the people she supervised — and taking very poor care of herself. She had stopped her alcohol abuse, but she had transferred her dependency to an old habit of abusing herself with food.

After a few months of our work together and a few weeks of AA meetings Peggy said, "I didn't know what 'selfcare' or 'taking care of myself' meant. I thought taking care of myself was goofing off or doing what I wanted to do. It never occurred to me that taking care of myself might be paying my bills, or cleaning my house, or refraining from eating unhealthy foods."

"Many people share your misconception. That's why it is necessary to do some selfhealing in order to start becoming selfcaring," I said.

"I've always had such a bad self image," Peggy said with a look of disgust on her face. "I'm not sure where it all comes from — the abuse I got as a kid from my older cousin or the fact I was fat when I was little. I've always felt inadequate — like I just wasn't enough."

I asked Peggy if she were willing to consider a different opinion of herself. She looked surprised that this was something she could change. I said, "Sometimes, before you meet someone personally, you may have a negative opinion of the person based on what others have told you or how the person looks on the outside. Once you get to know the person for yourself, you change your mind. So, how well do you know yourself to have formed such a strong negative opinion of yourself?" I asked.

She smiled, "Well, of course I don't know myself well at all. I've been spending my energy following rabbit trails that don't even lead to the rabbit."

I suggested to Peggy that we experiment with a way to access another part of her brain using a tool that I have always called Barry's Bodywork. I first learned it from Barry Stevens, one of my teachers.[4] I told her to close her eyes, go inside, and tell me where her awareness goes. She pointed to her solar plexus, and I asked her to describe what she found there.

"It feels warm," she said, "and I see something red, like a flame, a glowing flame." Surprised by how easily the images came, Peggy opened her eyes and said with some delight, "Hey, this is OK!"

I asked that she go back inside and become an observer of whatever happens and report to me what she notices. "Let's try an experiment." I said. "I'd like you to say, '*I'm* OK!' and notice what happens inside."

Peggy complied with my suggestion and then she said, "The warm sensation is still there but it's increasing, as though the flame is burning fuller. She paused to reflect on what was happening inside. "Now I feel full. You know, its like that feeling of satisfaction you have after a good meal."

"Let's try another sentence," I suggested. "Try saying, 'I am enough'."

Peggy again repeated the sentence I had given her. "Wow! Now the warm sensation is really strong. She repeated, "I am enough," and then the other side of her brain got it. "I *am* enough!" she said with delight.

As we finished our session together, I asked Peggy to turn around and notice the picture on the wall behind her. She was awed by Valerie Kneeland's picture (which is on the cover of this book) and the similarity to her own experience. There in the picture was the centered place that Peggy had imaged inside herself. As she studied the picture more closely, she seemed to be taking its image into herself. I shared with her that the image in Valerie's picture kept me connected to what selfcaring and selfhealing are really about. During the writing of this book, it was truly a picture worth more than a thousand words to me.

REFRAMING

Our mental attitude either contributes to or takes away from the spirit of what is happening in our world — like the frame around a picture. A powerful tool for selfcaring and selfhealing is to change the way we view a particular incident or situation — to reframe.

I remember a reframing experience which happened for me when the health center where I had recently started to work opened two new employee parking lots. This practical convenience soon became the object of much consternation as different individuals and groups began vying for particular spots in the lot nearest the staff entrance. I found myself getting caught up in the issues as others saw them until I stepped back and took a broader view.

The urban university I had recently attended had 25,000 students and 9,000 parking places, a dismal situation indeed. Looking at the present situation from the perspective (frame of reference) of my prior experience, I came to feel a parking place within a block or two would be a joyous privilege, and the brief walk a welcome price to pay!

THE HUMOR FRAME

Humor is an effective perspective from which we can make a reframing tool. This kind of reframing can change our perspective from negative to positive, from life-or-death serious to not-so-important after all. When we learn how to use humor to reframe, we are better able to maintain balance and sanity in work and family life.

The scenario of each person's on-going, ever-unfolding life experience can be seen as a personal situation comedy or a tragic soap opera. We don't need high paid writers to invent situations because, from moment to moment, we have the opportunity to create a soap opera or a situation comedy out of our life experiences. Let's do some role playing.

● ●

REFRAMING WITH HUMOR: AN EXERCISE

SCENARIO - (Soap Opera)

Take a situation in which you have felt aggravated. Remember when you found yourself getting in an uproar over some familiar or unfamiliar aggravation, inconvenience, insult, or injury (real or imaginary). Reliving that moment, now imagine someone asks you, "What's the matter?"

Pause! Breathe! Imagine a channel-switching remote control in your left hand. Click! Decide! On which channel do you want to play this particular scenario? Would this be a good soap opera?

Scene: "Transforming Your Aggravation" — Take #1

Decide which character you want to play and begin feeding lines to those persons (characters) standing nearby. See if they are able to improvise their lines based on what you are saying to them. If the lines the characters are speaking seem appropriate to the soap opera and if you find playing this role a satisfying way to live, see how far you can take this.

Consider renting a video camera and crew. You might make a demonstration tape (called demo in the industry). See if you can sell this act as a pilot to one of the major networks. Should you get turned down, consider independent syndication. If all else fails, make believe you are involved in afternoon reruns of your soap opera, and this will give you the opportunity to repeat this particular scenario in this particular manner on a daily basis.

SCENARIO - (Situation Comedy)

Scene: Transforming Your Aggravation — Take #2
Remember that situation where you were in an uproar as
above. Imagine someone asks you,"What is the matter?"
Pause! Breathe! Ask Yourself, "How would this matter
play as a situation comedy?" Select a comic character you
feel would do the greatest justice to your situation, and
play the scene from that vantage point.

You can call on inner guides in the guise of famous come-
dians you have known. How would Lucille Ball play this
part? How about Bill Cosby? Or one of the younger characters on his show? Traditionalists might prefer Charlie
Chaplin. (Practice his walk now.) How about Lily Tomlin's
Bag Lady, Trudy, with her Detroit accent? That poor woman
never does find any intelligent life in this universe!

Should you develop self-discipline enough in your real
life situations to choose the situation comedy routine
option more than several times in the same week (especially when the matter is the same old matter), you will
begin to discover that the Joker in the Sky (or whoever is
in charge of Humor Energies) will never let you run out of
humorous variations on any of life's themes.

• •

SUMMARY

In living a selfcaring lifestyle we are affected by habits
of the past, beliefs we have about ourselves and about how
others view us, and the feelings and attitudes we bring to the
helping situation. The dance of selfcaring in the mental
dimension involves. . .

Focusing on difficulties, barriers, and problems . . . . .

. . . . your body responds to this *negative picture* . . . .

. . . leading to your constructing even *more negative consequences*

. . . . resulting in your becoming . . . . .

. . . . DRAINED.

Or

Imagining a desired state . . . . . .

. . . . . your body/mind system responds, giving you . . . .

opportunity to *deal* with objections raised from any part of you . . .

leading to *elaboration* of the goal and *confidence* in a positive *outcome*

. . . . resulting in your becoming . . . . .

. . . . ENERGIZED.

And

Living in a *critical, analyzing frame of mind* . . .

. . . . creates *tension* in the body . . .

. . leading to *mental stagnation* and *lack of creativity* . . .

resulting in becoming . . .

. . . . DRAINED.

Or

Living *close to your imagining mind* . . . . .

. . . . allows *relaxation* in the body . . .

. . leading to *creative reframing, healing laughter, and solutions* . .

resulting in becoming . . .

. . . . ENERGIZED.

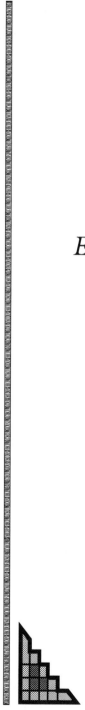

Every dance is a kind of fever chart,
a graph of the heart.

Remodeling and Reframing: The Emotional 8

> What I am feeling and how I feel about it are the essence of my
> experience, and as such are also the essence of both my
> development and my degeneration.
> Deane Juhan, *Job's Body*[1]

On T.V. I saw an amazing picture of a heart cell. Sitting in a dish by itself, the heart cell was pulsing visibly to its own internal rhythm. The camera panned back to show another heart cell in another dish nearby, also pulsing with its own rhythm. Their rhythms were quite different until they were placed in the same dish. Even before they touched, their pulsations synchronized into one continuous shared beat.

I remember thinking, "It's no wonder feelings are so contagious, our whole biological system is programmed to synchronize." Just being in the same room with somebody who is depressed or frightened or lethargic can mean those same states of feeling are evoked in us. That being the bad news, the good news of our vulnerability is that laughter, joy, and courage are contagious as well.

Feelings are the stuff of our kinesthetic senses. They are physical sensations not connected with sight, hearing, taste, or smell. Feelings are subjective perceptions of our own body sensations, and when a feeling is intensified it becomes an emotion. There are as many words to describe feeling states as there are words for the flavors of ice cream, but most are variations of a central few.

As people who do caring work, we must be able to connect with others at a feeling level without becoming emotionally drained ourselves. We must be able to identify and express our own feelings and able to allow others to express theirs. Avoiding feelings drains our energy, and being around somebody who avoids his/her feelings can be draining as well.

In the interest of our own selfcaring, we need to be clear about our own feeling states and learn how not to take on other people's feelings.

If, after spending time together, the other person (client, student, child, spouse, or friend) feels better and we feel worse, the situation has not improved any. The score just went from lose-win to win-lose, and only win-win counts.

ERRORS IN THE EMOTIONAL DIMENSION

There are two common errors in relation to feelings; not knowing what you are feeling, and using one feeling to avoid another.

Not knowing what we are feeling may come from years spent in higher education. There, intellectual processes are believed to operate without the information feelings provide. But feelings are essential guides for living. Our lives need to flow from our feeling values, and our feelings tell us what we care deeply about.

One psychologist I know described himself as "monolithic about feelings." Any sensation he experienced turned quickly into a mild to severe irritation which came across as anger. A lady whose children had been taken away from her through the trickery of her husband reported that she had been crying non-stop for days. I asked if she ever allowed herself to get angry and suggested it might be time to get mad.

These two examples show how, when one feeling is used to avoid others, the substitute feeling becomes extreme.

FROM ANXIETY TO EXCITEMENT

Mark was a young graduate student who had been participating in a movement group I was leading on his college campus. The men in the group had explored different kinds of movement from yoga, dance, tai chi, and systems of self defense. Emerging from these explorations was a realization of their over-reliance on logic and analytical skills while ignoring or avoiding feelings.

Mark had been struggling for several months, trying to come up with a topic for his dissertation in psychology. People had warned him that, since he would live with this decision for a long time, he needed to be certain to make the right choice for himself, now and for his future. One morning he reported the following breakthrough to the group:

"I was in the library looking through materials, trying to come up with a topic for a paper I had to write. I noticed that when I came across material on a particular subject I got a fluttery sensation in my stomach. When I put the material aside, the sensation left. Later, I came across something else related to the same topic, and the sensations returned.

All of a sudden it hit me. Instead of my usual anxiety, I was feeling mildly excited about that subject. Then I thought, 'Maybe this could be a way to select my dissertation topic!' I've concluded if I start out with a subject I have some excitement about, it will be easier to keep motivated for the long haul."

OTHER FEELING ERRORS

Feelings are contagious, and sometimes experiencing an emotion at an extreme level means that you have taken on someone else's feelings. A teenage girl whose family had recently endured a "polite" divorce told me she felt angry a great deal of the time. In addition to helping her express *her* anger appropriately, I worked with the more placid members of the family on allowing their anger. This way she didn't have to be angry for everyone else.

Selfhealing requires that we each be able to experience a full range of emotions because healing takes place through the full experience of the appropriate feelings. Feelings which have been driven too deeply within (stuffed) keep us from maturing into our real selves. Let's meet a man who came to me asking to get his body back. At first he reported feeling numb from the neck down and unable to identify or experience any feelings but vague discomfort.

GOOD GRIEF

I almost didn't recognize Jake in the crowded clinic waiting room. He seemed taller and more vibrant than when I last saw him a year ago. Jake had been in his late 30's when we started working together several years ago, but somehow he looked younger now than when we first met. This appointment had been requested by Jake for what he called an "emotional check in." He flashed a familiar broad smile as he extended his hand and energetically shook mine.

"There are some things you didn't tell me about getting my body back," Jake said as soon as the door to my office shut behind us.

"I wasn't aware of keeping anything from you. What have you discovered?" I asked.

"I've been having the strangest experiences lately, and I don't really know what to make of them. Maureen and I finally broke it off for good six months ago, and I'm doing real well. I've been able to see her kids and keep my relationships with them going strong. And when Maureen and I see each other, it's surprisingly pleasant."

I was remembering the painful sessions with Maureen and Jake as she attacked and he hid, frozen with fear and guilt. We worked to make the relationship more rewarding for both of them, and then finally the focus was on finding a way to end it.

"All the hard work you have done is paying off," I suggested. "You weren't able to put the relationship together, but it sounds as though you have found a way to release each other from cycles of blaming and feeling guilty."

"If anyone had told me three years ago that I would be able to feel this clear of Maureen, I would never have believed it," Jake said while gesturing with his hand up and down in front of his chest.

"You can take lots of credit for the work you have done to make this clarity possible," I said.

Jake smiled and said, "I remember when I first came to you, I couldn't cry. I would get angry or depressed, or what I called 'frustrated.' But that was just my way of getting ready to work myself up into being angry."

"And the two of you were quite a pair," I reminded him. "Maureen didn't know how to cry, either. She blamed you for not being in touch with your feelings and for somehow being responsible for her unhappiness. You would take in her bad feelings and carry them around for weeks."

"I remember the day Maureen and I were both here after you and I had done a bodywork session," Jake said. "I was able to express my pain to Maureen about the relationship not working."

I, too, was remembering that day as Jake described it. I said, "After you allowed yourself to cry in the individual session, you and Maureen were both able to experience and express your grief to one another. That was the beginning of your individual and collective healing."

Jake nodded in agreement. "But that is what's so confusing now," he said. "I went to a concert the other evening in that church on Elm Street with some friends. I was feeling at peace with myself and my life. The environment and the music were exquisite. I felt inspired by the whole experience until I noticed my eyes welling up with tears. I wiped my eyes, looked around carefully to see if anyone saw me, and then settled back into my seat. Before long it was happening again. You didn't tell me that when I learned how to cry I wouldn't be able to shut the tears off. And in public, too!" Jake said, half teasingly.

"You were touched by the music and the beauty of your surroundings. Tears aren't just for expressing grief and sadness.

Whenever something important is happening tears well up . It's your body's way of saying, 'Pay attention! This matters!' "

● ●

A FEELING QUIZ

Test your Emotional I.Q. with the following quiz.

Cover all of the columns in the chart below except column one titled "feeling." Now look down the list and ask yourself the following:

Which feeling(s) do you allow yourself to feel?

Which feeling(s) are missing from your vocabulary?

Which feeling do you have a tendency to get stuck in?

Which feeling do you have trouble allowing someone else to express without taking it on?

Uncover the other headings in the chart below. Describe your own subjective experience of each of the feelings listed.

Next note the suggestions of things to do and the description of some of the physical changes that may be occurring in your body.

FEELING	SUBJECTIVE EXPERIENCE	PHYSICAL CHANGES	THINGS TO DO
Fear	rigid stillness, shallow breath, inner chills	parasympathetic nervous system activated	keep moving, get support, express unexpressed feeling
Anger	tight chest, increased energy, stomach discomfort	stress chemicals activated	take assertive action, reframe as not serious, make creative expression
Anxiety	shortness of breath, sweaty palms, muscle tension	lactic acid produced as waste product	change breathing, reframe as not serious, laugh
Joy	warm sensations, internal massage	increased oxygen to blood, tension relieved	make creative expression, hug someone
Depression	lump in throat, labored breathing	endocrine and immune system supressed	grieve a loss, make creative expression

Ecstasy: A Special Emotion

One reason to take special care of ourselves is that there are some positive experiences in life for which we will need our energy — one such experience is ecstasy. Not often on the list of usual emotions, some people believe ecstasy is a part of our birthright as human beings. Not exclusively erotic, ecstasy is a powerful emotion of rapturous delight. Each generation of young children seems to discover anew the ancient secrets known to the whirling dervishes and Sufi dancers. Do you remember, as a young child, laughing and giggling, turning and turning until you fell down, and then getting up to do it again? Or perhaps you remember rolling down a hill in the soft grass, discovering a path to altering your consciousness and experiencing ecstasy.

Ecstasy is achieved by...
Approaching slowly from
a place of stillness
when you have committed
yourself to an exploration of
total openness to your own
and to others' ebb and flow.

Allowing alternating rhythms,
you move towards synchronizing,
synchrony with all parts of yourself
as well as with the universe.

Containment is necessary in order
to allow excitement to build,
until the ecstatic movement,
the moment of truth,
when we are able to allow
total surrender!

Each time is the first time,
for we are born again
with each complete and total act
of surrender!

Balance In Caring And Selfcaring

Most of us caregivers are sensitive to other people's feelings. In fact, this sensitivity can be a fault and a serious barrier to our own selfcare. Meet Sally, a nurse-manager in her mid forties who wanted to learn to set limits with a grown son and to be supportive to her mother who was ill with cancer. As the "mother in the middle" Sally was often pulled in opposite directions, having trouble taking care of herself in the midst of competing demands.

LESSONS OF THE MOTHER BIRD

"I'm close to exhaustion," Sally said. "The responsibility with mother's illness has been overwhelming these past nine months. And here I am trying to finish my degree while working full time and dealing with a 24-year-old son who lays around the house all day."

Sally breathed a huge sigh of relief as she began unloading some of the concerns she had been carrying around for the past months. As an only child she had been a wonderful daughter to her mother, and interactions related to her mother's illness had brought them even closer.

"So you have been helping your mother to die, and now it looks as though she is going to live longer than anyone expected," I said after getting more background on the subject.

"I guess that's a big part of it," Sally said, concluding with another labored sigh. "Right now though, I feel more concerned about my relationship with my son. I just had a fight with him, and I feel horrible. He hasn't worked in seven or eight months, and I feel I'm not helping him by allowing him to live there without looking for a job."

Over the weeks and months of our work together, Sally was able to discover how she took on other people's feelings. As we worked to heighten her kinesthetic senses, she noted the tension she created in her body when dealing with the feelings of her family members. When her mother was depressed about her illness, Sally felt tension around her heart and worried that she may have caused her mother to feel that way. After all, she had been wondering to herself how long she could sustain the caretaker role. When her son was angry with her, Sally felt tight in her shoulders and stomach. She asked herself what she had done to contribute to his anger. She had been involved with work and school as well as with her mother. Maybe he needed more time with her.

Sally told me later that the turning point for her came after an image of a mother bird had come to her during one of our sessions together. While she was in a state of relaxation, I asked her what advice the mother bird would give to her if it could talk to her in English.

Sally answered, "I see the mother bird in the spring, getting food for her young. She chews it, even partially digesting it before giving it to them. By summer the mother bird teaches the chicks to fend for themselves, pushing them out of the nest to fly on their own. The mother bird's message is, 'There are many phases to nurturing, many styles to the different seasons of our caring.'"

It took lots of practice, but Sally was able to stop taking on other people's feelings and to consider her own feelings in her relationships with her family.

"I felt very invigorated when I finally realized I could still feel good about myself, even when my son was acting like a jerk!" Sally said proudly. "And, since I am not in charge of my mother's happiness any longer, I think she appreciates the freedom to have a down day or two without my taking it on and trying to fix it."

HEALTHY ANGER

Anger can be a constructive emotion, but in my family nobody knew that. People expressed what I thought was anger, arguing, swearing, screaming — I still remember the screaming. I used to think this meant we had permission to be angry until I realized that our expressions of anger were followed by guilt and shame.

I now understand that we had confused anger with rage. What we were expressing was rage which is old, previously shamed anger. We weren't able to deal with the immediate situation that called for anger because of old, unresolved issues which had become rage. When people are stuffing their anger this often leads to raging later. When anger is respected and honored, important issues can be dealt with.

Anger is a healthy emotion and, as with most other feelings:

> Avoiding anger makes you sick.
>
> Repressing anger makes you sick.
>
> Expressing anger when you aren't honoring it
> leads to shame and guilt, which makes you sick.
>
> Denying anger makes you sick.
>
> Holding on to anger as resentment makes you sick.
>
> Confusing rage with anger leads to lack of control,
> which leads to discounting of your anger
> (more shame and guilt), which makes you sick.

An Ode To Anger

Anger is my truth, my life's spark.
Anger is my fire power.
Anger is the power to be, to become,
to make happen, to resolve.
Anger is my connection
to the electric universe.

Storms clear the air,
cleaning smog and cobwebs
out of the atmosphere.
Light follows thunder, revealing
clarity in stark edges of the
moist dawn.

EXPRESSING ANGER HEALTHFULLY

How would our lives be different if we could greet each others' anger as a life spark, a powerful connection to the electric universe? Learning to honor our own and other people's anger is not easy. Perhaps we should form the "Society For The Expression of Healthy Anger." We could practice expressing anger without hurting ourselves or others. We will need to be careful not to take ourselves too seriously, since anger does not have to be grim or ugly. Prerequisite movements for society members to perfect might include the following:

Stomping - Flamenco dancers do it while clapping their hands and shaking their castanets. People in the north woods do it to keep warm, to get the snow off their boots, to celebrate their connection to the earth. Stomping is a way to define boundaries, to clarify meaning. "This is where I stand. This is where I'm coming from on this issue."

Growling - Animals do it, like puppies at play. Sometimes we play too rough. It's a way to let the other person know, "You are going too far. Back off, don't take me for granted."

Spitting - Young boys do it, after much practice, in contests with one another. It is useful for underlining and otherwise punctuating important points in your argument. Women, due to cultural constrictions, suffer from spit deprivation and may need to practice privately until they develop the skill to hit their intended mark. Fair fighting rules demand that spitting is not a body contact sport and must not focus on population centers nor be done into the wind.

Chewing - People usually do it with food, tobacco, or gum. Domestic animals prefer bones, leather, and rubber balls. Since we are dealing with the most flexible joint in the body (the jaw), care must be taken these movements do not result in self harm. After chewing on your anger issues for some time, it is important to move to other, more expressive methods to release the anger energy and save your teeth, TMJ joints, and jaw, face, and neck muscles.

Punching - Cowboys, James Bond, and other cultural heroes do it on T.V. Since nobody really gets hurt, these performances mislead people into thinking that this is not a potentially lethal activity. Truth is, punching is for punching bags, and for pillows, sometimes while wearing protective gloves.

THE SOMA TWINS ON EMOTIONS

Let's check in with Touchie and Feelie about feelings and get their suggestions on dealing with our emotional dimension.

Feelie volunteered first. "Most people spend way too much time avoiding feelings or holding on too long to a feeling which, though unpleasant, is familiar. And when there is a continual repetition of the same feeling, other feelings are usually being avoided."

"Some avoidance of feelings comes from the fact that families and cultures have lists of approved and forbidden feelings," Feelie added.. "Some families do not allow expressions of anger, while others allow little else. In some countries like the United States, men are discouraged from crying, and grieving is considered a private matter. In other countries grief and mourning are expressed publicly in elaborate rituals. Men and women flagellate themselves and march through the streets to the sound of the funeral dirge."

"As far as the body/mind is concerned," Touchy says, "feelings are transient signals and expressions of inner needs and values. Tears often accompany one's letting go emotionally and physically. Feelings also provide information about what is happening in the environment and what direction to take."

Feelie adds, "It is possible to pick up the feelings of someone else, especially if that person is not in touch with his or her own feelings. The key to selfcaring here is to note the information you are getting from your own visceral sensations. If your stomach is grinding, and you can't identify anything that is happening with you, ask the person you are with to check inside themselves. If the signal belongs to the other person, let it go on through you."

"There is a vicious cycle that becomes activated when we hold on to or avoid certain feelings," Touchy continued. "Anger activates stress hormones, and it increases adrenaline and other chemical secretions harmful to our bodies if continued over a long period of time. People can become 'hot reactors,'[2] as Paul Pearsall describes in his book, *Super Immunity*. When activated repeatedly, this heightened state, produced by adrenaline, can become as addictive as any other psychoactive drug."

Feelie agreed and added, "People don't have to drink to get high. They can get high from their own brain chemicals generated by rage. Women in our culture are more likely to get hooked in a vicious cycle related to depression, becoming 'cool reactors.' If a life situation leads to a feeling of helplessness, biochemical changes take place in the brain. Norepinephrine, which is produced in the central nervous system, is depleted. This accentuates feelings of depression which further depletes norepinephrine, which — you guessed it — leads to more feelings of depression. And all of this affects the immune system and the type of diseases people are likely to exhibit."

"So, what needs to happen," said Touchy, "is to interrupt (or reverse) the cycle. Physical movement (exercise, dance, yoga) all increase the production of chemicals which contribute to a sense of well being. People can contribute to their own selfcaring by participating in activities to reverse the downward spiral of negative emotions."

"One problem I see," Feelie said, "is that people tend to think of feelings as pleasant or unpleasant, pleasurable or painful. This doesn't work too well, because then people try to hold on to or recapture pleasurable feelings and avoid what they are afraid will be painful feelings. A better way to think of feelings is whether they are of the productive or dead-end type."

"Holding on to any feeling," says Touchy, "will become dead-end because the system has to shut down to some extent. But the negative emotions pose special difficulties. Fear, panic, guilt, shame, and repressed anger all activate the stress system and inhibit the immune system. Laughter and the positive emotions boost the immune system, increase circulation, and provide an internal massage to the heart, lungs, and stomach!"

Both of the twins looked triumphant as they delivered the message, "It is better for our bodies, minds and spirits to cultivate the positive emotions, and to learn to interrupt the vicious cycles of negative emotions. We do this by taking care of the business of our life that has attracted or created them, and then moving the negative emotions through and out into the universe."

"Developing a strong sense of humor," said Feelie, "may be the most pivotal element in selfcaring and selfhealing, particularly for the folks who do the work of caring for others."

Lightening Up With Humor

Since feelings are the stuff of our experience, taking responsibility for our feelings means taking responsibility for our life. Just as a glass can be seen as half empty or half full, we have a choice: to focus on the dark or the light, the disheartening or the enlivening aspects of our experience. Humor is a vehicle which gives us that choice. We can choose humor, not just to cheer ourselves up or to deny our experience of difficulties, but to bring about a balance for our selfcaring and selfhealing.

Developing a sense of humor gives us the choice of looking at things from a lighter side. Humor disarms aspects of a situation (or of ourselves) which may have taken on more importance than they deserve. Even if you think you don't have a sense of humor, you can learn.

- Do you forget the punch line when you try to tell a joke?
- Were you noted in your high school year book as a "heavy thinker"?
- Or did you learn firsthand the hard lesson that it isn't fun to be the butt of a prankster's ridicule?

Do not despair, at least not until you have read further and learned how to perform comedic-tragedy. One thing to keep in mind as you attempt to break the shackles of your humorless past; you have a great advantage working for you. Since no one, perhaps even yourself, expects you to deliver a humorous response, your next joke has been set up by your usual serious facade.

I remember the response my dad, a quiet, serious man, used to receive from friends and neighbors whenever he would say something funny. His most powerful ally, the punch to his punch line, was the element of surprise.

• •

Rx For Humor Building

Now for actions on your own behalf. Just as you can change your diet and eating habits, you can begin to develop a humor habit. Laughter and play can feed your spirit as well as your immune and endocrine systems. If you have decided to make humor a key part of your selfcaring/selfhealing plans, here are some actions to take:

1. *Exaggerate!* Almost anything becomes ludicrous if you do it big enough or dramatic enough or fast enough. What is your tendency? Are you serious? Determined? Scattered? Do it more.

   • Place the back of your hand on your forehead and rise to your full height, head tilted slightly backwards, face to the sky. Picture yourself as a damsel in distress, the star of your own melodrama. (If you weigh 250 pounds and wrestle for a hobby, this will work even better.)

   • Oldtime silent movies seem funny partly because they are speeded up, causing the movements to be jerky. Enliven monotonous, dreary tasks by performing them in old time movie style, just for the fun of it.

   • Speak with an accent around friends, the phonier the accent the better. Picture horns or wings on the people you must be around in a difficult situation. Imagine, at a stressful meeting, place cards in front of each participant with the names of famous heroes and villains. (Try comic strip characters for variety.)

2. *Play the Polarities.* Opposites are often humorous when placed together.

   • Make a ceremony out of it! Mix ultra-formal and sloppy casual, (sneakers with formal wear, a baseball cap with your suit) Learn to dance back and forth between opposites. This may, on occasion, make it possible to find the elusive middle.

3. *Find Some "Partners in Crime."* Have you ever been to a joke-athon? You probably talk about current events, sports scores, or problems and difficulties with friends and family at home or colleagues at work. Why not share the funny things, and get practice in remembering and telling jokes. Telling jokes, like laughing, is contagious. Once someone starts off with a joke, others are reminded of jokes they have heard. Creating a place to tell jokes is a big help in remembering them, as well as a great way to learn new ones.

   • Clip cartoons and paste them around the house or work place. Send them in the mail to friends when you don't have time to write. In the midst of junk mail and bills, a cartoon is a welcome, loving message.

4. *Change the Medium!* T.V.'s Marshall McLuhan said that the medium is the message, so change the medium. Instead of saying it, make a picture, or sing it.
   - Draw a billboard, wear a button. If you and your situation were a statue, what would the caption read?
   - A picture's worth a thousand words, so put one in the place where you often get too serious, by the phone or over your bathroom mirror. This might cheer up the face looking back at you first thing in the morning.

5. *Reframe.* You know the expression, "When life gives you a lemon, make lemonade." Since there are no losses without gains, no joys without pain, humor can help us see the good that can come out of difficulties. In what situation would a particular experience be an asset? Maybe it's for the book you are going to write when your life gets interesting enough.
   - In front of a mirror, practice retelling a tragic event from your past. Intersperse the spice of humor as you elaborate the tale. Change the name of the central villain until you can tickle your funny bone. For example, if the man who "done you wrong" is named Dick, Dick becomes "Dicky," then "Sticky," then "Icky." If you are still having trouble smiling, put them all together. Every time you come across his name, as the plot thickens, refer to him as "Sticky-Icky-Dicky." If Linda left you in the lurch, let her be forever "Linda Lurch" or "Lurching Linda" in the memory modules of your mind.

● ●

SUMMARY

In living a selfcaring lifestyle we are affected by habits of the past, beliefs we have about ourselves and about how others view us, and the feelings and attitudes we bring to the helping situation. The dance of selfcaring in the emotional dimension involves. . .

Ignoring or *denying* bodily sensations ·········

affects *ability* to receive and process kinesthetic information ···

········· leads to inaccurate perception of self and others ·

resulting in *negative* emotions of fear, depression, and resentment.

Carrying around stored negative emotions results in ·········

····· becoming DRAINED.

OR

Attending to bodily sensations·············

affects ability to *allow* emotions to emerge from body ·······

········· leads to being able to *act* on emotional messages

by making creative expression, gaining insight, ·········

··· reframing with humor or taking assertive action ·······

····· results in becoming ENERGIZED.

I would only believe in a God
who could dance.

Renewing and Restoring: The Spiritual

9

> The balanced life of spirituality is reached when we comfortably
> can hold together opposites.
> Leo Booth, *Spirituality and Recovery*[1]

Sometimes our caring work doesn't have the outcome that we
intended. Sometimes we take on too much of what belongs to another,
wounding ourselves in the process. And there are times when, to
renew and restore our spirits, those of us who help others need help
ourselves.

WHO CARES FOR THE CAREGIVER?

"You and I are different, Sheila," Lois told me as we were
finishing up our work together at the hospital. She had been a
patient there for the past four months, and, though we had
done some beautiful work together, I had my reservations
about the safety of her being released at that time.

"You have taught me a great deal," Lois continued, "and
I have always felt that you really cared. But you have been
teaching me how to accept life on life's terms, and I don't want
that. If I can't have life on my terms, I don't want it at all," she
said firmly.

I remember the feeling I was having during that
conversation. It was as though someone had both hands on my
spine and were twisting it in opposite directions, as if wringing
out a beach towel. Lois had taught me, more than anyone else
ever had, the importance of taking care of myself, the importance
of knowing and respecting my limits.

It wasn't yet noon the next day when I received the message
that Lois had ended her life. Through the sense of shock,
horror, and disbelief, my husband and I reached out to each
other. We had worked together with Lois for many months.

Within minutes, we reached out to some colleagues at the clinic. We formed a circle together in one of the offices and prayed — for ourselves, for Lois, for her family and friends, and for the other caregivers who had worked so long and hard with her.

Less than five minutes later, a staff member asked me to come into the group room for a moment. There, amidst a room full of singing people, was a cake with birthday candles! As I caught my breath, I thought of a saying I used to have hanging on my office wall: "Choose life, every wonderful, terrible, delightful, terrifying moment of it!"

A HEALING RITUAL FOR THE HEALERS

Lois's parents wanted to thank the hospital staff for all that they did for their daughter. In the midst of their own pain, they wanted the staff to know that they realized everything that could be done for their daughter had been done. This need initiated the idea of a memorial service for Lois at the psychiatric hospital so that all those who had cared for her could participate.

During the service, Lois's father shared an important message for Lois's doctors, nurses, therapists, and technicians, and for all of us who work to help others. He began, "Friends and family members have been asking us, how this could happen after Lois had been in the hospital so long and so much had been done for her. Our answer is that if Lois had had cancer and had received all the most advanced treatments, she could have died anyway. If she had had a heart attack, she could have had a triple bypass — the most advanced technology — and she could have died anyway. The fact is, we all are only human, and what that means is you can't save them all. Most people understand this when the problem is primarily physical, but the same is true for mental, emotional, or spiritual problems. You are not God."

The chaplain ended the brief service with an important message for everyone, especially those of us who work with ill and troubled people. He reminded us of the last words of advice given by Socrates to his friends, just before he drank the hemlock. "Practice dying."

THE SOMA TWINS ON THE SPIRITUAL DIMENSION

I wasn't sure this was something the twins would want to deal with, but they had been so helpful in describing how they interact with the physical, mental, and emotional dimensions, I invited their comments. I told them that our scientific culture hasn't wanted to deal with the unseen world of the spirit. Priests and minister-types are allowed to discuss such matters, but when anyone else mentions the spiritual, it seems to trigger theological arguments or fears of voodoo and black magic.

Touchy began, "I'll never understand how *seeing* got to be so important for you folks. Nobody sees sound or heat waves, or atoms or germs with the naked eye, yet scientists are quite comfortable with these unseen phenomena."

Feelie joined in. "Restricting the spiritual dimension of life to churches has slowed down the process in understanding what it is to be truly human, and what life is really all about."

I reflected, "I notice when I do body-oriented psychotherapy with someone, when all the parts of the person are connected up and energy is flowing freely between all the parts, they seem more than the sum of their parts. Spiritual themes emerge suggesting to me that *holiness* is really *wholeness*.."

Touchy added, "When people are in that self-transendent place they are able to carry out their sacred missions."

"And what is that mission?" I asked, more than a little curious to see how he would describe it.

"Each person's mission is to become who he or she truly is," Touchy said. "All primitive cultures used the body to experience the spiritual self. Through dancing, the use of chants, becoming aware of the breath (all ways to still the mind), the body becomes a kind of antenna, tuning in to subtler and subtler levels. When this happens often enough, the person finds direction and purpose, a place in connection to all of life, and one's own path."

"Realizing where they have been, they know where they are going as well," Feelie said.

I remarked, "I remember a woman I worked with who was feeling very stressed by her unhappy marital situation. As she began, in her body, to let go of the struggle to find an answer, she heard a line from a Beatles song: 'Let it be, let it be, there will be an answer, let it be.'"

Feelie smiled in recognition, "That is one of the songs that my inner wisdom sings to me, too."

I remember another client who received a powerful spiritual message by tuning into her body. She described herself as being in a situation of great stress at her job. She was being mistreated by a co-worker, and, during a session to mediate their differences, she experienced a loss of hearing in her right ear. During a break in the session, her hearing returned. When the session resumed, her hearing difficulty returned. She had done a lot of prior work on paying attention to her body and decided that, in this situation, some part of *herself* was trying to tell her something. As she listened carefully to her own inner voice she heard, 'Be still, and know that I am your God.' What turned out to be right for her was *not* to go along with the agreement that the people in her office were trying to arrange for her.

Both Touchy and Feelie were smiling and nodding agreement by this time. "You are describing the stillpoint," Feelie said.

"Yes," said Touchy. "Spiritual reality exists at the point where all things converge and connect. And you can get to that place when you really need to by having practiced one of the disciplines of quieting the logical mind and heightening your sensory awareness. You can recognize the spiritual messages because they always take into account opposites; in other words, *everything*."

At this point, I asked Feelie to describe the stillpoint in her own words, but she assured me that T. S. Eliot had already done that much better than she could. She recited the following poem with deep emotion in her voice:

At the still point of the turning world. Neither flesh nor fleshless;
Neither from nor towards; at the still point, there the dance is,
But neither arrest nor movement. And do not call it fixity,
Where past and future are gathered. Neither movement from nor
     towards,
Neither ascent nor decline. Except for the point, the still point,
There would be no dance, and there is only the dance.[2]

AN ARMY OF ANGELS

It was the beginning of a workshop on selfcare, and the leader, Ilana Rubenfeld, told the following story of an experience she had had in Brazil in the early seventies.

"I had been in a great deal of stress in my personal life and working very hard in my professional life. I began experiencing an odd symptom, a numbness in the third and fourth fingers of each hand. I reasoned that if I'm doing something I really love, passionately, and I am getting sick or wounded, something is wrong. Since I was traveling in Brazil at the time, a friend suggested that I go to one of the traditional native healers for whom Brazil is famous. The message to me from the native healer was, "You are only one little person! There are too many who need your gifts. For what you are doing you need an army of allies in heaven, an *army of angels!*"

A PATH OF PAIN

Later in the workshop, a 69 year old man named Leonard asked to work with Ilana. The difficulty that he presented was a recurring pain in his back, which had been chronic for many years.

"I don't let it stop me from doing what I want to do, but I can't help wondering what my life would be like without it," he said.

Since retiring from his job as an agency director, Leonard has enjoyed the fruits of his labors, living a full, active life. He and his wife have traveled whenever their volunteer and community responsibilities allowed.

After gently touching his back, Ilana asked, with simple curiosity in her voice, "When do you first remember having the pain?"

"When I got out of the army in '45," was Leonard's matter-of-fact answer.

While continuing her gentle touching, Ilana asked, "Did anything special happen at that time?"

At this point, Leonard was in an easy state of relaxation, enjoying the experience of touch and talk. From this place, his answer seems almost lackadaisical, "Nothing much. Just the usual stuff that happens in war."

The workshop participants responded with laughter as Ilana smiled and echoed his sentiments, "Nothing unusual, eh! Just regular war stuff, huh?"

After a brief pause, Ilana continued, "Is there anything that happened at that time that still feels unfinished for you? Something that may still be sitting there in your body that we could help you to let go of?"

Leonard responded with a blank look on his face. "I don't know," he said.

Ilana encouraged him, "Start with anything," while she continued the gentle touching of his back muscles. "Just start with any regular old war stuff."

"I was in charge of troops. My troops liberated the

concentration camps." He remained emotionless, a reporter of facts.

A shift in the mood of the group became evident as the group responded to more than the facts. I was seated across the room taking notes and moved closer to Ilana to offer moral support. As Ilana continued her supportive touch she made an effort to take care of herself in relation to this difficult theme. She whispered to me, "Sheila, just wipe me off."

Sitting behind Ilana, I began moving my hands in the air, several inches from her body. This movement, which we sometimes refer to as an "energy wipe" created a flow within the energy field around Ilana and Leonard. By continually repeating the movement which went from the base of Ilana's spine the length of her body and upward towards the sky, my positive energy assisted Ilana in discharging the negative energy surging from Leonard through her. For all present, this kinesthetic reminder suggested it is possible to direct the tension and energy of Leonard's releasing up, up and away from our own bodies.

As Ilana continued working with Leonard, I continued my port de bra (dance of the arms), moving the energy upward to the heavens and sometimes downward into the earth. Leonard's story unfolded, coming out of the releasing in his body. He related losing family members in the concentration camps.

"Both my parents, my brother, sister, uncle and cousins. I lost my whole family in the camps."

My response inside was, "I didn't think the U.S. military would send a Jewish person to Germany during Hitler's reign."

Ilana asked Leonard to describe his family, and he began to remember and relive pleasant times when the family members were together. Leonard talked about skiing with his father and other family members in Austria when he was growing up.

As he spoke of the pleasant memories, the muscles of his back continued to soften. It seemed clear that he had not recalled and reclaimed these joyful, happy memories since his experience at the camps.

"So," Ilana encouraged him, "You can remember skiing with your father and the others, the wonderful warmth and joy of the fun you and your family had together. These experiences belong to you, and you can go there anytime you want to remember all the wonderful gifts that your family gave you — all the gifts that are a part of you now."

The Message In An Image

From the movement that I was doing, I began to get an image of a guardian angel. As my arms moved in a flowing fashion behind Ilana, I remembered the pictures of guardian angels on the walls of the Catholic school I attended as a child. From this sensation of flight I began to get an image of lots of angels. I remembered Ilana's earlier story about the Brazilian healer, and, reacting to Leonard's story, I whispered to Ilana, "I know who your angels are! There are six million of them at least. All the people from the concentration camps! They are surely an *army of angels!* "

As Leonard completed his work, in the peaceful reverie of family remembrances, he joined the group with the look of a child just waking from a nap. Ilana played a tape of a full orchestral version of a Viennese waltz. I remember thinking, as everyone in the room, including Leonard, began dancing, that dance therapist Marian Chase, the founder of dance therapy, was right, "Waltzing cures everything!"[4]

Leonard's work continued to reverberate throughout the rest of the week-long workshop, though not much was said in the group until the last day. As we began bringing our time together to a close, workshop participants, although of different ages and nationalities, began dealing with the universal themes ignited for them by Leonard's work.

Contagious Feelings

Members of the workshop expressed gratitude to Leonard for allowing them to witness his letting go of his long-carried pain. This atmosphere of appreciation changed when it was a young German girl's turn, and she began to cry.

"I have so much shame! I feel so much guilt," she said, with a heavy accent. "I know it makes no sense. I wasn't even born then, but it was my people that did those terrible things."

The group members sitting near the young woman reached out to her, putting their arms around her and supporting her. I moved behind the woman and the group members comforting her, and repeated my "guardian angel movements" as I had done with Ilana when she was working with Leonard. At this point I heard a voice from deep inside me that said, "No more victims! No more!"

No More Victims

Peopleworkers! Be aware of the lessons in Leonard's story:

> **If we store our reactions to horror and atrocity in our bodies, we keep the atrocities alive, interfering with our own vitality!**

and

> **Working with people who are troubled or in pain is hazardous work. It takes a power greater than ourselves to keep us from taking in and holding on to toxic realities.**

Selfcaring Skills In The Spiritual Dimension

As I remember my experience with Leonard and Ilana and the young girl from Germany, I realize it was a turning point in my life. In that situation I saw clearly the exact nature of my vulnerability as a helping professional and my need for assistance in taking care of myself.

The human condition means that we are all wounded and likely to become overwhelmed by the harsh realities of our own or other people's pain and suffering. Some people choose to deny harsh realities in order to protect themselves. For those of us who have been victimized and treated unfairly ourselves, anger about our own experiences can draw us like a magnet to take on more than we can handle.

SORTING AND SEPARATING, the first selfcaring skill, needs to be done from a spiritual perspective. Some things only God understands. I do not know why bad things happen to good people or how nations can be wiped out by people who believe they are doing the world a favor. All I can ask is, what does this mean for my own life? What am I here for? My prayer for myself in those moments is that I be able to stay present to the person in need of my help so he/she may learn the lessons from his or her own experience.

Using the second skill, LETTING GO, began when Ilana assisted Leonard in letting go of the pain of his past. The rest of us had to **let go** of our reaction to his situation. Negative energy is magnetic and some members of the group had special vulnerability to the theme of Leonard's pain. Jewish members, including Ilana, had to avoid taking on the victim pain. The young woman from Germany needed help in letting go of the shame of her German ancestors. Everyone's selfcaring choice: to remember the positive, mourn our losses, and join in the waltz.

The spiritual dimension is made up of PARTNERSHIP POWER. No one acts alone. Ilana used the power of the group as a healing circle around herself and Leonard. She asked for help from me, and I brought guardian angels from my childhood and a suggestion that she send the pain to what the Brazilian healer called *"an army of angels."* Adding the spiritual dimension to our work and life means recognizing our connection to others, to one another, to those who have gone before us, to the positive energy in the universe, to whatever name you give the God of your understanding.

The fourth selfcaring skill, STEPPING BACK, is illustrated when Ilana encouraged Leonard to step back from the ending of the lives of his family members to appreciate the gifts they had given him *during* their lives. And, for the group members and leaders, there was a balancing of the pain and negativity with the positive memories and the mutual support we gave to one another. STEPPING BACK enabled us to witness one man's pain while being supported by a caring community. From this emerged a commitment to live in such a way that we no longer become or create victims.

To EXERCISE CHOICE in the spiritual dimension we must remember that, as human beings, we are capable of heinous crimes as well as noble deeds. While facing the negative, we have the choice to despair or focus on the positive lessons learned. If we do not take into ourselves the pain and atrocities of the past, we are free to create a better world for ourselves, for one another, and for those who will come after us. By way of taking care of myself and facing up to my own experiences of atrocities I wrote the following poem:

A RECIPE FOR FORGIVENESS SOUP *
*When it appears that bad things happen, or have happened, to good people,
consider the following recipe for forgiveness soup.*

Take at least:

*two parts **breath**, (as in keep breathing!)
one part **movement**, (as in keep moving!)
one part **release**, (sometimes called prayer,
as in "let go and let God!"
Send it to the Army of Guardian Angels!
(That's what that heavenly host is for!)
Stir slowly all ingredients while humming your favorite lullaby.
As the pot starts to boil, season silently with smiles.
You will find your solution beginning to bubble with delight!*

*(*When used as a trail mix, this soup will lighten your luggage and
backpack. Especially recommended if you plan to travel through rough
terrain or scale high places.)*

• •

EMBODYING THE VALUES OF THE SPIRIT

When we leave behind the hustle and noise of our busy lives, we often discover our external life situation doesn't match the values of our spirit deep inside. This incongruity can be scary and difficult to deal with. One way to connect more fully with your spiritual self is to identify more fully with your own value system. The following activity can help in the selfcaring, selfhealing journey of becoming and living, the values of your spirit.

1. After a brief time of inner quiet, identify a universal value that is important to you. It could be honesty, humility, courage, generosity, justice, love... to mention but a few.
2. While remaining in a relaxed state, allow an image to emerge that represents the value you have selected.
3. Identify with this value by saying or writing, "I am (here name the value)."
4. Identify with your image by becoming that image. For example: Experiencing yourself as a bird to represent freedom, as a warrior to represent courage. Notice your feelings in the role of the person or object representing your treasured value.
5. Ask yourself, "Have I known the opposite value?" Write about that.
6. Ask yourself, "How do I deal with these values in my present life?" (Note: A variation which works better for some people is to work with the image before the verbal message.)

Let me offer the following example, working with one of the values closest to my own stillpoint, the value of justice.

FROM INJUSTICE TO JUSTICE

When I was involved in a difficult, unequal relationship, I found myself using a lot of energy just maintaining my sense of self respect. I was kept occupied continually confronting the other person's manipulations and mistreatments of me. Periodically, the relationship would even out and work mutually well for awhile— until the next storm, when I couldn't see any remnant of our past discussions or agreements. I worked on this relationship for several years because I loved the other person and I was dedicated to the work we were doing together. And, after all, nobody's perfect.

Finally one day, as I was meditating, I discovered that I had a soul hunger for justice. As I made this discovery I knew that this hunger had been there all of my life and that I had a pattern of being in close relationships where a just balance was impossible to achieve. For justice's sake (which is to say, my own sake) I had to leave what I loved. I finally realized that love cannot exist without justice.

For us caregivers — and helping professionals, and caretakers of our children and our elders, nurses to the sick, teachers of the young, counselors to the troubled — justice requires that all parties flourish, and in that balanced equation lives love. It is said that luck is a lady. Well, meet the lady Justice.

You've seen her standing in her Grecian robes, erect and tall. A blindfold covers her eyes and she is centered within so as not to be distracted by appearances. Under one arm she carries the book of knowledge acquired through many ages. In her left hand she holds a scale to weigh both sides of the issues in conflicts and disagreements. Since she is blindfolded, Justice cannot read the scale or become distracted by the appearance of things. She cannot read the expectations and opinions of others in their facial expressions or body postures. Justice must sense, from her own center, the subtle differences of weight on each side of the issue. Her own kinesthetic sense tells her the exact configuration, the exact point in time and space when the scales are in balance.

From that place of centeredness — that stillpoint — having let go of everything, Justice makes decisions that are right and fair and just. Staying in her own center, a place of clarity and love, Justice acts that all things may flourish in the fullness of time.

It may be helpful to understand what justice is *not*.

Justice is *not* what people are ready to accept.
Justice is *not* what people are comfortable with
at a particular point in time.
Justice is *not* what people "think" is fair and just.
Justice is *not* what people have made a case for in the past.
Justice is *not* what I can persuade people to agree to.

I AM JUSTICE

I am Justice!
I have taken my turn.
The sting of painful small injustices,
Insults, taunts, and teasing putdowns,
Sarcastic insinuations.
I've been slapped, shunned,
Misunderstood, wrongly accused.

I am Justice!
I have paid my dues.
Watching powerlessly
Other people's mistreatment.
Tall teacher humiliating my
trembling classmate.
Strapping father
beating my little brother.
Scolding mother talking
through clenched teeth.
Feeling sorrow, guilt,
embarrassment, and shame.

I am Justice!
I know the pain of
large scale inequities.
Help Wanted Signs:
"No niggers (or Irish,
or women or Mexicans)
need apply."

I am Justice!
I have done my homework.
Fine tuning my breath,
Standing up for myself,
Joining hands with my sisters,
Singing, dancing, and
Letting go of the pain.

The Spiritual And The Elements Of Selfcaring

In the spiritual dimension, attention is focused on the deep, inner self. The intention is for healing, for making whole. When we are coming from a place of balanced centeredness we experience our connection to all that has gone before, to fellow travelers who share our journey, and to those who will follow after. Our attitude, once we involve the spiritual dimension, is one of wonder, appreciation, gratitude, and curiosity. These qualities of being in tune with what is happening spring from the experience of life as a gift. We no longer live in "hurryup" time but slow down to tune in to subtle levels. Spending time in altered states of prayer and meditation, we delight in small and simple things.

Movement in the spiritual dimension involves surrendering completely to each phase of the dance including the places of stillness.

Nourishment for our souls comes from communing with nature, surrounding ourselves with beauty and order in music and the visual arts, and participating in rituals which reinforce and express our values. *Support* comes from a loving community, from connection to ancestors and other spirit guides, and from the God of our understanding. *Pleasure* and *Play* form connections between our child selves and our spiritual selves. *Humor* and *Rest* enable us to keep a clear perspective, not taking ourselves or the events of our lives too seriously.

● ●

SUMMARY

In living a selfcaring lifestyle we are affected by habits of the past, beliefs we have about ourselves and about how others view us, and the feelings and attitudes we bring to the helping situation. The dance of selfcaring in the spiritual dimension involves. . .

Movement in the spiritual dimension . . .

involves *surrender* . . .

into a place of *stillness* . . .

leading to a discovery of connection . . .

to people and values important to becoming our *true selves* . . .

resulting in moving from being DRAINED to becoming ENERGIZED.

Act Four

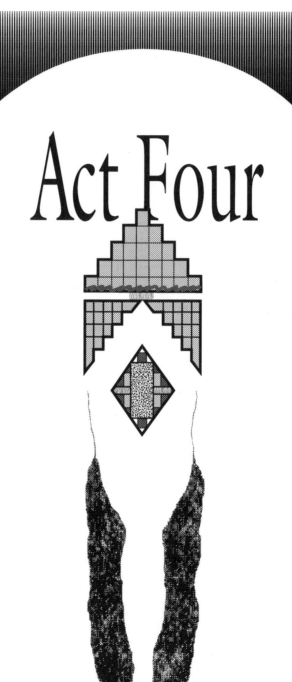

The
Dance

*D*ances are always a central part of community ceremonies and celebrations.
In order for caregivers not merely to go through the motions or mark
time (as in rehearsal) but to dance fully with joy and exuberance, we need the
support of a loving community. Learning to design and perform rituals,
we create opportunities to come together and celebrate at work and with our
families. When our rituals are about peace and we join hands in
dances which celebrate who we truly are, each person flourishes....and
the world becomes a better place.

The dance - it is the rhythm of all
that dies in order to live again:
it is the eternal rising of the sun.

Reconciling and Recreating Your Life

10

Let there be peace on earth, And let it begin with me.
Sy Miller & Jill Jackson

The setting was a women's international peace conference, and a dark-skinned woman in ceremonial dress had taken the microphone. "The world doesn't have time to wait until everyone in the privileged countries achieves inner peace," she said in a powerful voice tinged with sarcasm.

"And I don't have time to wait for peace in my life until the politicians achieve world peace," I found myself saying to myself in a quieter voice.

The fact is, we human beings don't do well living in war zones. Peace may be a *prerequisite* for solving our personal, family, and global problems, not a *consequence*. Our psychobiology functions best when we can stay out of our survival mode. And we get along better with others when everyone can avoid pressing his or her panic button. Our wounds from prior hostilities need an environment of peace in which to heal. To become truly selfcaring and selfhealing means, in the end, to become a peacemaker.

Since both inner and outer peace are the best-case scenarios for people and all other living things, one would expect most everyone to be working to accomplish this glorious end. But peacemakers are not in over-supply in any country around the globe. Cities have trouble locating qualified peacemakers, churches and work organizations often run them off, and many families struggle to survive without a single peacemaker in residence.

It has been suggested that peace will not prosper until we clear up some small misunderstandings regarding the nature of peace. With all the excitement generated by war, border skirmishes, and police actions, people have a tendency to think of peace as boring by comparison. Many people haven't yet discovered a peacetime equivalent to the good feelings generated by war-torn comrades sticking together to fight the enemy. Many people have difficulty marshaling their forces or conserving their resources unless threatened by someone they see as a fierce competitor. It's little wonder most of us haven't a clue about where to begin to achieve one's own inner peace.

In the psychobiological model presented by this book, peace is the re-creation of balance and harmony among parts of ourselves, with our past, and with the people in our work and home environments. When we rely only on what others seem to need, or how it has always been done in the past, we experience anything but inner peace. Our job responsibilities may pressure us to spend more time at work while the needs of family members may be calling for our services. In the face of such competing demands, in order to achieve inner peace, we must find a way to consider our own needs along with the needs of others. Selfcaring and selfhealing are central to bringing about the reconciliation necessary for achieving inner peace — and eventually communal and global peace. As we practice the selfcaring and selfhealing actions in the four dimensions described in this book we will find ourselves becoming peacemakers.

Once we achieve peace (not to be confused with boredom), we become engaged in a vigorous dynamic dance. In the process each of us brings forth his/her very best. Once experienced, our whole system prefers peace. However, peace is difficult to maintain. How can we continue to hold peace in our hearts as we rush through our days? Pushing ourselves to accomplish today's "to do list," we oppress ourselves. When we are tired and drained from overextending and overdoing, we take it out on others. And when we are criticized? How peacefully do we handle people whose views deeply challenge our own?

As we continue practicing the skills of selfcaring and selfhealing while staying in connection to those we care about, we continually recondition ourselves for peace. As conflicting and contrasting parts of ourselves are integrated into a consistent, harmonious whole, we develop integrity. In fact, *integrity is the evidence that integration has taken place.*

By living our lives in a selfcaring, selfhealing way we take responsibility for bringing all aspects of ourselves into alignment. When physical, mental, emotional, and spiritual dimensions are in alignment, balance and harmony are achieved.

BUILDING A PEACEMAKING COMMUNITY

Consider our connections to one another; this balance and harmony can not be achieved alone. We need each other. We affect one another. It is in peacemaking community with others that we each become who we truly are. Let's look at one of the most effective tools for building community, that of creating our own rituals. And let's remember — just as it is said the job can create the person, or people become what they do — together we create the community, and then the community creates us.

What words do you associate with the word "ritual"? Participants in a workshop on selfcare suggested the following words: *ceremony, transition, change, rite of passage, solemn, religious, continuity*. Rituals are events designed to make experience special. My favorite definition of ritual came from one of my teachers, Anna Halprin: *"Rituals are what love does to experience."*

Rituals are part of the fabric of our lives. They are so woven into our everyday life that we don't recognize them for what they are — rituals. Think about how we honor one another annually, on the anniversary of one's birth with cake and candles and singing of the Happy Birthday song. Or think of particular family rituals such as setting a special place at the table for an honored guest or the particular way in which Christmas presents are exchanged each year.

Graduation and marriage are important times of change in people's lives, often celebrated with elaborate rituals. These ceremonies have elements of strong traditional symbols which is probably why, in times of social change, people begin writing their own ceremonies. Their hope is that, by reflecting the new order of things, old symbols can be reclaimed and institutions can be renewed and revitalized.

To the casual observer, communal rituals may seem to belong more to primitive cultures we have only read about, but our modern age has its share of ritual. Fourth of July parades commemorate a link to our historic past. In fact, most of our holidays are observed with ritual of one kind or another. Awards dinners, whether held at the local school or televised to the entire nation, celebrate outstanding accomplishments in sports, theater, and music. Some people have suggested, with the advent of television satellite transmission, the entire world has become a global village. Through the magic of technology we are now able to participate, at least as spectators, in the political, sporting, and religious rituals of peoples throughout the world.

Some rituals are solemn and religious. But even secular rituals have strong spiritual elements because rituals represent invisible and indescribable aspects of life. Rituals can be public or private, elaborate or simple. They always involve action, symbols, and other elements of good theater. Rituals are designed to involve and transform the audience as well as the people performing them.

Ritual can have its dark side. Rituals can become either a blessing or a curse. A family reunion may become an occasion to gossip about the people who couldn't, (or weren't invited to) attend. A Friday night ritual get together with coworkers can degenerate into an occasion for continually complaining about the boss.

On a larger scale, many of us remember the horror of Jamestown, when hundreds of members of a religious community went to their deaths in a ritual of mass suicide. Members of neighborhood gangs have been known to carry out heinous crimes as part of group rituals or rites of passage. Hitler's political rallies used ritual to build a community which would uphold the practices and principles of the Third Reich, replacing traditional ethical behaviors.

Because something can be misused doesn't mean that we should avoid it altogether. It does mean that we need to look carefully at the rituals we are already participating in. Do these experiences support our health and well being? It may look like love, but is it killing us with kindness? One organization I belonged to had wonderful gatherings where people sang and swayed together, but the members had no real say in the organization. Ultimately, participation in the rituals of this organization kept us all as children, relying on a single leader.

Taking responsibility for our lives as true grownups means refusing to participate in rituals that do not empower us and contribute to our own and the community's greater good. It means learning to use ritual, to create rituals which build the kind of community we need for our mutual selfcaring and selfhealing.

A Simple Ritual For Peace

At a professional meeting in New York several years ago, a man led the group in a thirty second ritual which he had received in Germany from someone who got it from the Gandhi Foundation in India. I began teaching it to my staff and starting off each of my therapy groups with it. I noticed the powerful effect it had on me and the other group members and the way in which it set a tone of peace and reconciliation.

A year later I was asked to participate in an international women's peace conference in Dallas, Texas, and I brought the ritual to that occasion. Each day we opened the proceedings with the ritual. It was performed from the stage by women of different nationalities, each saying the words in her own language. We made hundreds of copies of the ritual, and the women took it back to the 65 countries they represented. Even as you read this, perhaps, they are sharing it with their families, friends, colleagues, and neighbors. Remember the soft drink commercial which sang about teaching the world to sing "in perfect harmony"? We can hope this type of activity is getting us in condition for peace.

● ●

A Universal Greeting

This Universal Greeting from the Gandhi Foundation is easy to learn. Place this book where you can read it and yet have both hands free. Think of someone with whom you need to have a reconciliation. Imagine yourself saying the words which follow and making the gestures to that person. Or perhaps you need to start off in front of a mirror, sending this message to yourself. As you say the words, perform the gestures: they are based on universal sign language and move beyond the barriers of verbal languages. Allow yourself to experience the movements as a graceful dance. Later teach this greeting to a group of people who are interested in working together peacefully.

I OFFER YOU PEACE
(Face palms forward, elbows bent)

I OFFER YOU FRIENDSHIP
(Cup hands palm to palm, elbows bent)

I OFFER YOU LOVE
(Draw hands forward from heart)

I HEAR YOUR NEEDS
(Cup hands behind ears)

I SEE YOUR BEAUTY
(Cover eyes with hands, then uncover)

I ACKNOWLEDGE YOUR FEELINGS
(Arms cross chest, fingertips to shoulders)

MY WISDOM FLOWS FROM A HIGHER SOURCE
(Right arm moves in an arc from behind the head to meet
 upturned left palm at chest level, fingertips forward)

I SALUTE THAT SOURCE IN YOU
(Palms together in prayer position)

LET US WORK TOGETHER
(Fingers interlocked as two-handed fists pointed upwards)

The Ritual Of The Cornbread

I was first introduced to the power of ritual because of some cornbread. While I was living in the eastern part of Nebraska I was coordinating a project for human service workers in the western part of the state. The goal of the project was to learn more about the Native American and Mexican American cultures and, however modestly, to improve the system for providing human services to better meet their needs. I asked a Native American professor of fine arts to accompany me to the project site as a guest speaker for the course I was organizing.

The woman, Gaylyn, told me she would be willing to participate if I could get her some cornbread. She explained that on the date we were discussing she would be coming off her monthly fast. According to her native traditions, fasts are broken by cornbread. When asked to help, the Native American women from the region where the class was held were eager to be helpful regarding the cornbread. They seemed concerned however, about the kind of cornbread that would be appropriate. As members of a different tribe than Gaylyn's, they were aware that each tribe is likely to have its own recipe for this important staple. When I asked Gaylyn she laughingly said, "Any kind will do, just so it's corn bread."

Gaylyn and I traveled by plane and then car to the hotel and workshop site. Time seemed to go by quickly as we got to know one another better. She was learning more about me and the project I was coordinating, and I was learning more about her and her life and culture. That evening, after Gaylyn's presentation, several women came forward with the important cornbread. As we thanked them, I noticed they seemed honored to be asked to provide it.

Gaylyn and I went back to the quaint little hotel in the center of town where we each had a room. As we were saying good night, Gaylyn surprised me by asking if I would like to join her in her room to witness her ritual. I remember experiencing the same feeling of gratitude as the women who had baked the corn bread. I felt honored — and a little scared that I wouldn't know how to act.

A dozen years have passed since that night in her hotel room, but tears come to my eyes each time I remember it. She had a pipe and some other sacred objects, and I remember her praying out loud and allowing the smoke to trail into each of the four directions. Many details of what she did and said are hazy to me now, but I will never forget the feelings of blessedness that I had as I witnessed her ritual.

She prayed for the project, that it would serve the native people. She mentioned the women who had made the cornbread. And then she prayed out loud — for me. She understood, as I did not, that my being in that leadership role as project coordinator would transform me. She asked that I be given the courage to listen to the people and to the part of my inner self that was created to serve. The ritual ended as I dried my eyes and we broke cornbread together.

We spent several other days together later on, working on the project. I remember a post card from her...and later a Christmas card I sent, but we lost track of one another long ago. I remember telling my students how close I still feel to this woman after all these years. It's as though we are relatives. I have come to understand that such is the power of ritual. Though we shared many thoughts and ideas, told each other stories of our backgrounds and cultural experiences, it was the ritual that made us sisters forever.

DESIGNING MY OWN RITUALS

After my experience with Gaylyn's cornbread ritual, I began to develop a new appreciation for the power of ritual. Native Americans, in living with ritual, set a strong example of how to appreciate the sacredness of all of life and how to bring that idea into our everyday consciousness.

DESIGNING A WEDDING CEREMONY

Like many couples married in the sixties and later, my husband and I designed our own wedding ceremony. We bought a book that explained the meaning of the symbols and practices of a traditional wedding. This way we could decide what parts we wanted to include in order to affirm certain values — and what needed to be eliminated as not representing what marriage meant to us. Since we were from different religious traditions, we purposefully included aspects of each to signify a blending of our two traditions. Because of the differences in our family backgrounds, no one in either family was particularly pleased with our marriage. Family members on both sides came to the ceremony with much trepidation, taking each of us aside in turn, making suggestions and requests regarding the ceremony. Warnings of impending doom were also communicated should we do (or not do) certain things.

Fortunately, the minister who was to preside had not only given us free rein ("Just write out what you want me to say,") but he had told us: "In my experience, once the ceremony happens, the struggle is over and no one remembers the fears." He seemed to be saying that the ritual would work its own magic.

I'm not sure we believed him, but we proceeded as though we did. In our wedding ritual the family members danced and sang together. And when the inner circle of the dance (my family) joined with the outer circle (his family) a marriage of two very distinct families was accomplished as well. My daughter sang, my sons poured the wine, and everyone danced and cried.

One family member said the ceremony stayed with him for days. "It was so powerfully emotional," he said. I still do not understand how, but, in effect, all relationships were different from that day forward. Had we known that would happen, we might have arranged to have the ritual sooner, rather than waiting several years for the courage to do it.

A CAREER RITUAL

Many years later I stumbled into designing my own personal ritual. This was not for a traditional occasion like a wedding, but rather on an occasion that normally would not be celebrated at all. And I wasn't really thinking I would *do* the ritual, I just wrote and thought about it, and this gave me great strength and pleasure through a difficult time.

I had traveled to New York to work on a writing project. Just before I left Texas my university boss (and mentor of six years) told me that he had changed his mind and would not be supporting me for tenure. This betrayal was a total shock to me and to everyone involved, since I had gotten an 8 to 1 vote from colleagues in favor of my tenure request. I arrived at my hotel room, set up my computer, and as I typed the words, "A Healing Ritual," I began to heal.

I visualized the ritual; I saw the scene, the people, the place. I heard the music. I began typing a description of what was going on inside my head. As the words flowed out from my fingers, feelings of relief moved throughout my entire body. My spirits lifted as I laughed at the satire of a funeral I was designing for my university career.

In the months that followed I handled the treachery that continued to be played out by rewriting and rereading my ritual. This was a wonderful way to step back for a broader perspective and to keep a clear distinction between the death (murder, really), of my career and my own continuing aliveness. Later it became evident that, for my own healing, I needed to actually perform the ritual. I sent the following invitation to my friends, family, and professional colleagues:

Iatreia Institute for the Healing Arts
in cooperation with
The Mini Mouse School of Social Work
and
The Center For Women Who Work Too Much
Presents
SHEILA K. COLLINS'
TRANSFORMATION OF A CAREER: A HEALING RITUAL
Saturday, September 5, 1987
7 p.m. Reception to follow ceremony

The actual text of the ritual is included in Appendix A following this chapter as an example and an act of encouragement to all of you who have (or will) experience career dissolution, betrayal by colleagues and friends, or simple disappointment upon the death of a dream.

DESIGNING YOUR OWN RITUALS

Career situations are not the only type of situations which can benefit from ritual. Life-changing events such as divorce, retirement, relocating or moving, to name a few. In any situation of major life change, a ritual can be a powerful tool for selfcaring and selfhealing. Consider the following worksheet to help you collect the various elements needed for your own ritual.

● ●

RITUAL PLANNING WORKSHEET

1. Identify the *situation* in your life which calls for constructive change.
2. Describe yourself in the *old* situation or state.
3. Describe yourself in the *present* situation or state.
4. Describe yourself in the *new* situation or state that you are moving towards.
5. As you move into this new phase of your life, list what you intend to:

Leave behind   Take With   Develop New

<----------   ----------   ---------->

6. **Resources For The Ceremony**

People - Consider the people you want involved and what roles you want them to play. You may want to allow a time for people you have invited to say a few words as is done at memorial services, or, in a lighter vein, at roasts. Give clear directions. Remember, "This is your life!" This is your party, and you can cry and laugh when and if you want to.

Readings - Think of scenes from literature, classic myths, or fairy tales. The main idea here is to tap into the universal theme of your situation as it may have been treated by classical writers. This will help you to see your personal tragedies and triumphs from a larger perspective.

Music- Select anything from opera to musical comedy to folk to country to popular. They will all work, depending on the metaphors you want to use. Singing is a wonderful way to involve certain people — or the audience as a whole.

Symbols/Objects - Think of archetypical objects, objects that carry strong meanings in all cultures: fire, water, light, bells, drums. A filing cabinet and a bonfire were used in my ritual. Gaylyn used a pipe and other objects sacred to her culture's traditions.

Movement- Think of a way to represent the movement that you are making in your life. Rituals are always about moving from one situation or state of being to another. Processions and dancing offer ways for the audience to become participants with you in your ritual.

7. *The Score* (On a single sheet of paper describe what you will do in each phase. Include time and space considerations for each phase, the beginning, the middle, and the end.)

RITUALS IN THE HOME

It isn't necessary to wait for big events like weddings or funerals to experience a ritual. Events in a particular family member's life can be a time to pull out your ritual planning worksheet. Mother's promotion at work, a teenager's receiving his/her driver's license, a youngster's overcoming failing grades at school — these are all occasions that many families celebrate now. Planning a ritual just makes it more conscious and purposeful.

Short, less formal rituals can have a big effect on family life. One family I knew had the philosophy that each child desires some time each week to be an "only child." They arranged a weekly walk, a trip to the store, or a talk on the porch swing for each child alone with dad and then time alone with mom. When children are small this special time can happen at bedtime. Remember, one definition of ritual is "what love does to make experience special."

Events which affect the whole family such as a move to another state, or a divorce are not usually marked by ritual. Yet it is in situations of dramatic change such as these where rituals can be powerful tools for healing both individuals and the family as a whole. If it fits with your religious values, you might consider asking a minister or priest to formally bless your new house or participate with your family in a ritual of forgiveness to help the family move through a divorce.[1]

WORKPLACE RITUALS

Think about the organization where you work, and begin to notice that rituals already are going on there. How are staff members' birthdays celebrated? What about coffee breaks? Company picnics or the Christmas party? How are people rewarded for outstanding performance or honored for years of service? More than likely there are rituals that have sprung up over the years for these and other special occasions.

Make sure these practices reflect the values you want to encourage in yourself and others around you. One woman told me, "At our company, whenever we do something good, they feed us!" She was referring to the staff luncheons and breakfasts and award banquets that made it very difficult for her to maintain a healthy weight. All the rituals at her work place involve sweet and fattening food.

A man I knew had to leave his job for health reasons because all the in-service and training events involved extensive "happy hours" with the booze flowing freely. High performance was rewarded by many toasts to the honored guests, and excessive overworking was encouraged as the norm in demonstrating loyalty to the "company store."

On a more positive note, one workshop on selfcare for executives of social service agencies generated a lively discussion of how these bosses structured time for positive work place rituals. They used special occasions for enjoyable time together to build skills in teamwork and collaboration.

Take the example of a new staff member or student trainee joining an established group. The meeting begins with a question each staff member is invited to answer. The question is different each time, but it always has something to do with each person's relationship to his/ her work. The question might be, "When did you first know you wanted to do the work you are now engaged in?" or "Who is the person who most influenced your work and how?" Or "How is your behavior at work similar to, or different from, your behavior in the family in which you grew up?" While providing the newcomer with an interesting way to get acquainted with the staff, this ritual gives oldtime staffers a new look at each other.

A New Beginning

An owner/manager of an insurance agency enlisted my help in designing a ritual for the opening of his small agency's new offices. The company had been through a major reorganization and many difficult physical and emotional changes. He wanted to recognize what the agency and its employees had been through in recent months, to celebrate the new office, and to look forward together to an exiting and challenging future.

A memo was sent to employees announcing this special event and enlisting their participation in the planning. Each person was asked to fill out the following worksheet.

1. In making the move to new offices, list anything you hope to leave behind.
2. List anything you want to be sure to bring along.
3. What are you especially looking forward to at the new location?
4. Do you have a specific contribution you would like to make to the festivities? Describe.
5. In the spirit of improving the office environment, what "rules" would you like to suggest for the agency?
6. Are there any "rules" that you feel have been operating in the present office that you would like to see eliminated? Describe.
7. Name any music that you feel would be particularly appropriate for this occasion.

Material from these worksheets were compiled into "Leaving Behind and Bringing With - A Litany," recited with the theme from "Raiders of the Lost Ark" playing in the background. The following new rules of the house were constructed and sung as in a Gregorian chant.

Rules Of The House

There will be no smoking, chewing, spitting, and drinking
of alcoholic beverages on these premises.

Employees and associates will check their bad moods
in the parking lot and smile upon entering the front door.

Employees and associates will notify the
establishment of their whereabouts whether in or out,
or when due to return to the office.

Language at this agency shall be at all times fit
for polite company, not offensive to gentle men,
ladies, and innocent minors.

Using all proper forms, work submitted by 9 shall be out by 5.

Employees and associates, remember:
Reality is not always the way *you* see it,
so respect others' points of view.

Warning: Should these rules be broken, serious consequences
shall befall the offender, as the establishment is
henceforth serving notice — No More Nice Guy!

THE FINALE

Caring for others is a hazardous occupation, made less so when we have learned to care for and heal ourselves. The state of the world can only get better when we learn to use what life is presenting us as fuel for our fire, breath for our song, and energy for our dance. Rituals can help us celebrate our connection to one another and build the community of support necessary for each of us to take care of ourselves. Like the chick emerging from its shell, the snake shedding its skin, and the caterpillar becoming the butterfly, selfcaring and selfhealing require transformation to mature adulthood, all the while nurturing the ancient child within.

So often we stop ourselves from joining in the dance. Another participant at the international peace conference in Dallas showed me how to courageously break through reservations and unreasoned fears and this led to an unexpected and transforming finale.

I presented a peace dance in the lounge of the student center where the conference was held. Conference participants were seated around the room informally as artists from different countries performed for them and for one another.

As I was in the middle of my dance, a dark skinned woman I did not know jumped up from her seat. In ceremonial dress she joined me for a most joy-filled duet. I did not know her country or her language, but a sense of deep understanding passed between us as we danced together spontaneously. Later I learned of the conversation which occurred prior to our dancing together.

The woman in the colorful dress said to her companion as they watched me dance, "Oh, I feel so inspired to join her."

Her companion said, "You can't do that. You're too fat!"

Disregarding her companion's protest, the woman, recognizing a shape that I was assuming in my dance, said, "That is like yoga; I know this. Of course I can!" and she proceeded to act on her inspiration by joining me in my dance.

And you, too, can join in the dance by creating and performing your own rituals and transforming your own life. Include personal rituals of selfcare which balance the essential elements of movement and stillness, work and play, pleasure and pain, and experiences of connection and solitude. Practice the skills of selfcaring and selfhealing by doing your own sorting work, letting go and surrendering and don't forget the duet, building and using partnership power. Sometimes, at those crucial points, step back for a broader perspective, and always and continually, exercise choice. From the stillpoint of our inner world may each of us transform our caring dance from one that drains us to one that gracefully expresses who we truly are.

EPILOGUE

● ●

The dance changes the dancer. The practice of the technique changes the dancer's body, the rehearsal changes the dancer's mind and emotions, and the performance changes the dancer's spirit. Caregiving done as a dance, wholeheartedly with one's body, mind, emotions, and spirit, transforms the caregiver.

And sometimes this transformation comes late in one's life, after other careers have ended. I learned of this first hand from my own parents. During the three years or so of my mother's terminal illness, my father became her caregiver. She had been a nurse — always a caregiver of others. Driving in the limousine to the cemetery we family members tried to name all the different people mother had taken into our house. She collected stray, needy people like children sometimes collect stray, needy animals. Mother had always worried about my father and how hard he worked. She believed, and even had us convinced, that she would end up taking care of him.

It seemed a strange role reversal. Dad, the engineer, became my mother's nursemaid. Dad, who rarely took even an aspirin himself, kept track of mother's many medications and told her which pills to take and when. And since Mother was unable to carry out her usual caregiving chores, Dad stood in for her with friends and neighbors. Though not a Catholic, he started going to Mass with mother every week, something he never did when we were children. Nothing in his early life growing up on a farm, or later on, in his training and experience as an engineer, had prepared him for this new career as a caregiver.

I didn't see it on a daily basis; I lived too far away. But when I came to visit I would see the changes in them both. My mother, growing sicker and more dependent, struggled with the unfamiliar and often uncomfortable role of receiver rather than giver. She would fight him, determined to preserve some semblance of her former independence.

The changes in my dad were pronounced also. He gained weight, and often looked tired. But he seemed softer, happier to see us, and more talkative. I noticed that his eyes would moisten with tears when he mentioned something that was important to him. This happened on the day I realized that the role of caregiver had changed him.

We were talking about the changes in the liturgy and how much better it was that the priest now spoke in English. He mentioned the blessing at the end, when the priest would usually turn to the congregation and say, "God be with you. Go in Peace!" One particular day the priest changed the wording of the blessing to "God be with you. Go and serve one another!" My father had tears in his eyes as he told this to me, and he followed it with a comment, said in his own unique style: "And baby, that's what it's all about!"

NOTES

●●●

PROLOGUE

1. Laing, R. D., *The Politics of the Family*, (N.Y, Vintage Books, Random House, 1969, p.31)

2. Maslach, Christina, *Burnout -The Cost Of Caring* (Englewood Cliffs, New Jersey: Prentice-Hall: 1982).

3. For more about the status of women's work see: Statham, Anne; Miller, Eleanor; Mauksch, Hans; editors, *The Worth of Women's Work, A Qualitative Synthesis,* (Albany, New York: State University of New York Press, 1988).

4. For an excellent examination and delineation of a caring ethic see Noddings, Nell, *Caring, A Feminine Approach to Ethics and Moral Education* (Berkeley, California: University Of California Press, 1984).

5. Selye, Hans, *The Stress of Life* (New York: McGraw Hill, 1978) *Stress Without Distress* (Philadelphia: Lippincott, 1974).

6. Seigel, Bernie, *Love, Medicine and Miracles* (New York: Harper and Row, 1986).

7. Alexander, F. M., *The Use of The Self* (New York: E.P. Dutton, 1932. Centerline Press edition, Downey, California, 1984).

8. Feldenkrais, Moshe, *Awareness Through Movement,* (New York: Harper and Row, 1972, 1977).

9. Rubenfeld, Ilana, "Beginner's hands: Twenty-five years of simple,"*Somatics* (Spring/Summer 1988), pp. 4-11.

CHAPTER 1

1. Soma is a Greek word which means living body and refers to the self sensing, internalized perception of oneself from the inside. See Hanna, Thomas, *The Body of Life* (New York, Knopf, 1980) or Hanna, Thomas, *Somatics*, (Massachusetts, Addison-Wesley Publishing, 1988) pp.5-7.

2. In spite of the Bible's positive reference to dancing (Psalm 150, "Praise the Lord with your dancing!"), some Christian churches continue to forbid dancing as sinful.

3. Timothy Leary and others began experimenting with drugs as a way to alter consciousness and learn more about how the mind works.

4. I am indebted to Ilana Rubenfeld for the notion of using the image of brackets to prevent past events from contaminating present interactions.

5. For expanded definition of a partnership model which involves linking with others rather than dominating others see: Eisler, Riane, *The Chalice and The Blade* (San Francisco: Harper and Row, 1987).

CHAPTER 2

1. This prayer was written by Reinhold Niebuhr and later made popular by members of Alcoholics Anonymous and other twelve step self-help groups.

CHAPTER 3

1. Poems were written by Ralph Caplan for Herman Miller Corporation's ad campaign to introduce modular office systems. Used with permission.

2. For more about the way interior design impacts our behavior see: Caplan, Ralph, *By Design,* (New York: St. Martin's Press, 1982).

3. Rubenfeld, Ilana, "Selfcare for the professional woman: Beyond physical fitness," *Women and Work, Selected Papers,1985* (Arlington, Texas: Women and Work Research and Resource Center, 1986).

4. I am especially indebted to the designer, Louis Nelson, for his discussion with me regarding the importance of lighting in the work place. See also: Venolia, Carol, *Healing Environments* (Berkley, California: Celestial Arts. 1988).

5. DeForest, Cathy, "The Art of Conscious Celebration: A New Concept For Today's Leaders", 1985, in *Transforming Leadership: From Vision To Results,* Adams, John, editor, (Alexandria, VA.: Miles River Press,1986). Used with permission.

CHAPTER 4

1. Title IX, the federal enabling legislation of 1972, states "No person on the basis of sex shall be excluded from participation in, or subject to discrimination under any educational program or activity receiving federal financial assistance."

2. Consultation to school districts took place under auspices of The Center For Co-Equal Education, University of Nebraska, Lincoln, funded by the U.S. Office of Health, Education and Welfare.

3. Examples of the slowness of the wheels of justice include the fifty plus years it has taken for reparation checks to be sent to the survivors and heirs of the Japanese American citizens incarcerated in camps during World War II. Closer to home, personally, is the class action salary discrimination suit, filed in 1974 and never settled, on behalf of women employees of the University of Nebraska.

4. For further information about Codependents Anonymous For Helping Professionals write to: CODAHP, Box 42253, Mesa, Arizona 85274-2253.

CHAPTER 5

1. This technique was inspired by R.D.Laing's *Knots,* (New York: Random House, 1972).

2. For more information about the Rubenfeld Synergy Method contact The Rubenfeld Center, 115 Waverly Place, New York, New York, 10011.

3. The programmed messages referred to here have been identified in the system of Transactional Analysis as the most common drivers, (motivators which "drive" a person to behave in certain ways). According to this theory, messages from childhood interfere with the person's ability to be inner-directed and supersede a person's meeting his or her own needs.

CHAPTER 6

1. Juhan, Deane, *Job's Body* (Barrytown, New York: Station Hill Press: 1987) p.19

2. Appreciation to Dan Millman for the five aspects of physical fitness. See: Millman, Dan, *Warrior Athlete; Mind, Body, Spirit*, (Walpole, New Hampshire: Stillpoint,1985).

3. Workshop leader in this example was Ilana Rubenfeld who is also an Alexander Teacher. For more information about the Alexander Technique see Alexander, F.M. (above in Prologue) or contact North American Society Of Teachers of Alexander Technique, Box 806, Ansonia Station, New York, N.Y , 10023.

4. Silverman, Julian, *Health Care And Consciousness* (New York: Irvington Publishers,1983).

5. Juhan, Deane, *Job's Body*, (see above) p.xxix

6. For a discussion of the anatomy of stress see: Nuernberger, Phil, *Freedom From Stress* (Pennsylvania: Himalayan International Institute, 1981), Chapter 2, pp. 35-74.

CHAPTER 7

1. Rossi, Ernest, *The Psychobiology Of Mind-Body Healing* (New York: W.W. Norton, 1986).

2. Gawain, Shakti, *Living In the Light* (San Rafael, California: New World Library, 1986).

3. Achterberg, Jeanne, *Imagery In Healing* (Boston: New Science Library, 1985).

4. Stevens, Barry, *Don't Push The River, It Flows by Itself* (Berkeley, California: Celestial Arts, 1970) and Gendlin, Eugene, *Focusing* (New York: Bantam Books, 1981).

CHAPTER 8

1. Juhan, Deane, *Job's Body*, (see above) p. xxviii

2. Pearsal, Paul, *Super Immunity* (New York: McGraw Hill, 1987).

CHAPTER 9

1. Booth, Leo, *Spirituality and Recovery* (Pompano Beach, Florida: Health Communications, 1985) p. 4.

2. Eliot, T.S., "Burnt Norton," *Complete Poems and Plays, 1909-1950* (San Diego, California: Harcourt Brace Jovanovich, 1950, 1980), p. 119. Used with permission.

CHAPTER 10

1. Musical resources for family rituals include Beethoven's "Consecration of the House Overture, Opus 124," and the folk song, "Bless This House."

APPENDIX

• •

GUIDES TO AID PHYSICAL SELFCARE

Most of us were not taught how to attend to the needs of our physical selves as a crucial part of our selfcaring. The following two guides are offered to aid some of the small but important decisions you will make which impact on your physical health and well-being, and therefore on your mental, emotional and spiritual self as well.

GUIDE FOR SELECTING A CHAIR

What kind of movement is the chair capable of doing? Since you may be taking this chair to different workstations and wanting it to accompany you through different tasks, flexibility and movement are imperative.

1. Can the chair be raised and lowered easily?

2. Can the back tilt or recline without raising the seat?

3. Can the chair move easily over the surface of the floor while you are sitting on it?

4. Will the wheels lock in place when you don't want the chair to move around the room?

B. What is the nature of the support the chair gives you? The major role of a chair is to support you in supporting yourself. As you sit in postures which are healthful and easy to maintain for extended periods of time, the chair should be a contributing ally and friend.

1. Notice the scale of the chair in relation to your size. Can you sit easily with your feet on the floor and without the front edge of the chair pressuring the back of your thighs?

2. Try out a seat with a saddle design. Like when you are riding a horse, these seats separate your legs so that you are sitting on your sitz bones. (These are the bones that seem to be tailor-made for sitting. Sit upright on your own palms and you will become familiar with them.) Note that this style chair comes in male and female proportions and celebrate the fact that at least some chair designers have finally taken into consideration that men and women are built differently.

3. Move the chair up to your work station. Does the back of the chair support you as you move closer to the work station? (This is partly related to the

positioning of the armrests and whether they will fit under the desk or work table.)

4. Can you adjust the back of the chair so it matches the contours of your back? Some models have a mechanism to insert air into the back cushion. This means that the chair conforms to the person sitting in it rather than the other way around. This feature is also available in the driver's seats of some new cars, especially helpful for people who do a lot of driving.

C. Keep in mind the cost of your chair. Remind yourself that you will pay now or pay later. Decide that you are worth an investment in support for your structure as you do your life work. If you are in a position to purchase chairs for employees, the same principles apply. The added incentive as an employer is that by providing supportive chairs for employees you can prevent paying later the costs of absenteeism and workman's compensation settlements.

SELECTING A PHYSICAL ACTIVITY

Ask yourself the following questions regarding any activity which is supposed to benefit your physical self. Does the physical activity:

1) Develop your awareness and enhance sensitivity to yourself and others?

2) Does the activity energize you? (Is it vigorous enough to help eliminate toxins from the body?)

3) Does it respect the realistic limitations of your life situation? Does it allow time to meet other needs of your life?

4) Does this activity consider any limitations you have from prior injuries? Does it work with, not against, your genetic build?

5) Does it reeducate and strengthen muscles?

6) Does it avoid producing injuries?

7) Does participation in this activity increase your ability to relax?

8) Does it provide challenge?

9) Does the activity feel fun and enjoyable most of the time?

APPENDIX B

MOVEMENTS FOR MENDING

I. BREATHPLAY

Taking control of your breathing is a powerful way to take control of your life. A colleague of mine, Ian Jackson, has written a whole book on this subject, but let me suggest one of his most powerful techniques, one he calls Upside Down breathing. This technique reverses what we normally do when we get anxious and try too hard. After some practice, this technique can be done standing, sitting, while driving a car or riding a bus, but we'll begin lying on the floor.

1. Begin by getting comfortable on the floor. Place your hands on your lower belly and press in as you exhale.

2. After you have exhaled all your air, release your hands and allow air to come back into your lungs automatically.

3. Next, actively press your lower belly again, expelling all your air.

4. Release your hands, and stay passive as the air rushes back into your lungs.

5. Appreciate that your job is letting go of the old air, and that new air comes to you automatically when you are able to make room for it.

II. *METAPHORICAL BREATHPLAY*

Ian and I have found the power of this simple breathing exercise to be greatly enhanced by adding imagery and the intention of healing as you perform the movements.

1. Think of something in your real life that you would like to let go of or eliminate from your thoughts and feelings.

2. As you breathe out, imagine that you are eliminating whatever you have selected in step 1.

3. As you relax to allow air to reenter, picture taking in to yourself something that you need more of in your life.

4. Keep an open mind to these new possibilities, and notice any changes in your life after a week or so of practicing these movements.

III. *POLARITY PLAY*

This is a wonderful way to escape the limitations of an either/or view of the world. Playing frequently with these possibilities will help you get unstuck and teach you respect for the wisdom of your own body.

1. Select two opposite (or what seem to be opposing) qualities. You may use tension/relaxation, giving/receiving, courage/fear, strength/weakness, or select selfcaring elements you are having trouble bringing into balance. (See list in Chapter one.)

2. Create a gesture or movement to represent the first quality you have selected. Perform this first movement.

3. Now create a movement to represent the second quality and perform this movement.

4. Moving in slow motion, perform the first movement followed by the second.

5. Continue moving back and forth between the two movements.

6. Notice if the movements change in any way as you perform them in this manner. Allow this to happen by simply following the movement and where it 'wants' to go.

7. Your reward for suspending any judgement or opinion that this is 'foolish' or 'doesn't make sense' will be that you will discover your body's way of creating harmony and balance in the physical dimension.

8. Reflect on what this information might mean in other areas of your life.

9. Thank your kinesthetic senses for their gift of wisdom.

IV. *MUDRAS - (RITUALLY SYMBOLIC GESTURES)*

A man goes to his priest, (rabbi, minister,) and reports his discomfort in no longer believing in the faith of his youth. He would like to become a believer again, but he doesn't know how. The spiritual leader gives him a simple prescription, "Each day assume the posture of prayer and behave as though you have the faith that you seem to have lost. We are built in such a way that we become what we do."

1. Assume a kneeling position. Place palms together in front of your body with fingers pointing upward.

2. Begin slowing raising your hands upwards towards the sky. Allow your face and neck to follow your hands.

3. When you have reached the extent of your range in this direction, slowly lower your hands.

4. When your hands have returned to the level of your heart, begin sitting back on your feet.

5. Bending from your hips, begin separating your hands and reaching out towards the floor in front of you.

6. Surrender your weight to the floor as you surrender your will to your Higher Power.

7. Stay in this place of surrender until you feel propelled from your center to move.

V. *TRY EASY!*

I am indebted to Al Chung-liang Huang for the inspiration for this movement for mending. A T'ai Chi master, Al is also a master at getting people to move with the quality of the chi (life force) without getting hung up in a perfectionism of doing the form correctly. The spirit of the ancient art of T'ai Chi is to playfully practice moving with a "try easy" spirit, challenging oneself to let go of any unnecessary tension. Try easy to make each movement as effortless and pleasurable as possible.

1. Stand with feet separated at least the width of your own shoulders.

2. Balance equally on both feet so that your body is positioned in the center of the space between your feet.

3. Soften your knees so that they bend slightly. (Remember, your knees are your shock absorbers and, when locked, they cannot operate for this purpose.)

4. Gently move the trunk of your body to the right and in a slightly curved angle, shifting your weight so that it rests on your right foot.

5. Move the trunk of your body gently in the reverse direction, through the center and to the left so that your weight is on your left foot. The path you are traveling is like a C turned on its side.

6. Repeat these movements, making sure that you are breathing to accompany the movement.

7. Now add movements of the arms and hands so that they accompany the rest of your movements. As arms move inward toward the center, inhale; as arms move outward, exhale.

8. Experiment with different arm movements, coordinating the hands and arms so they are together in front of your body when your weight is in the

center. Allow your arms to move out into space as you shift your weight to one foot or the other.

9. The quality of your movement should be like the graceful slow motion replay of televised sporting events. Some people use the image of moving through clouds, or moving in a weightless environment such as a space ship, or swimming underwater like scuba divers.

10. Continue these movements for two to three minutes, allowing the movement to change as you explore moving as effortlessly as possible.

11. As you are moving, notice any places in your body where you begin to have discomfort or tiredness. Imagine sending your breath to these places so that you may let go of any excess tension you are carrying.

Extra bonus -

12. After you are comfortable with this type of movement, add a message that you would love to believe deep in your soul. Repeat the expression as you perform the movements. Examples: "I am relaxing in the arms of the unfolding universe." "The world is unfolding in exactly the right way." "I am a valuable and precious person."

VI. *BOUNDARY BUILDER*

Peopleworkers need to be careful not to take in the toxic energy of complaining clients, hostile staff, blaming bosses, or pleading family members. One way to take care of ourselves is to boost our boundary system and practice building boundaries of protection.

1. Rub palms of your hands together.

2. Keeping palms facing one another, separate them slightly. Begin moving palms in relationship to one another until you can feel the energy or sense the space between them. (Some people experience temperature change or a sense of density in the space between their hands.)

3. With your hands, begin tracing an imaginary boundary for yourself in space, several inches from your body. You can strengthen this boundary by imaging a color and consistency of material. Remember that this boundary needs to be semipermeable to allow positive energy to enter and negative energy to leave.

4. Turn your palms outward and move this "space capsule" you have created so that it can expand as you stretch out in different directions. Make certain that you can move freely inside the area that you have defined for yourself.

5. Explore any place where your protective membrane may need extra fortification, (perhaps in front of your heart, or behind your back, or behind your knees). Fortify these more vulnerable places by imagining a thicker membrane around those places. Imagine sending your breath to those places as you move.

REAL LIFE APPLICATION

When you find yourself feeling drained in the presence of a particular person, remember this activity and imagine doing it in your mind's eye. Later, if you must deal with the person again, you may perform the entire movement series immediately prior to coming into their presence.

VII. *LETTING GO*

Giving up control, even the illusion of control is often difficult, and a great deal of the tension in our bodies comes from over controlling. Since most of us control with our heads, this movement is good practice in literally letting go of our heads. The hope is that mental, emotional, and spiritual forms of letting go will follow.

1. In a standing position, move your wrists as though you were shaking water off your finger tips. See how loose and "out of control" you can allow your hands to be.

2. Bending forward slightly from the waist, allow one arm to hang loose from its socket.

3. Experiment with allowing your right arm to be moved by the rest of your body. Try swinging and circular movements.

4. Resume a standing position and notice any difference between the shoulder and arm that has been moving and the other one.

5. Now allow the left arm to move passively as you bend slightly from your waist.

6. Return to an upright position and rest.

7. Standing with feet wide apart and bending forward from your waist, allow both arms to hang passively from their sockets in the center between your feet.

8. Turn your head gently, loosening your neck and allow your head to join your arms. Begin moving in this position, keeping your arms and head loose and free.

9. Resume a standing position and regain your equilibrium.

10. Swing your arms gently from side to side, and then slowly shift your weight to the left foot as your arm swing enlarges to the left, and both arms move in an arc as high as you can reach over your head.

11. Swing your upper body in an arc, leading with your head and arms through the hanging position to the other side. Your weight changes from the left foot to the right at the completion of the swing.

12. Repeat the swing from side to side several times, practicing the quality of surrender as you move through the hanging position that you started with.

VIII. *PARTNERSHIP POWER: SUPPORTING AND FALLING*

The expression, "he's not heavy, he's my brother," only works if we know how to lift another without hurting ourselves. This movement activity is done with a partner and will provide plenty of practice in ways to support another without hurting oneself. Then when it's your turn to fall, you can practice letting go and accepting support from another. I am indebted to Anna Halprin for this movement from her "Circle The Earth Peace Dance".

1) The supporting person stands behind the person who will be moving. The supporter places his/her arms around the mover just above the hip bones.

2) The moving person inhales and on the exhale, allows his/her head and neck to fall forward till the head is even with the middle of the chest.

3) On the next inhale, the moving person rises back to an extended position, standing.

4) Meanwhile, the supporting person behind offers just enough resistance to the one moving that he/she feels supported in the fall.

5) The mover repeats the falling movement on the exhale, this time going farther, till his/her arms touch the floor. (The mover should be able to let go and actually fall and be caught by the supporter. The supporter can do this if he/she matches the breathing of the mover.)

6) The mover repeats the falling movement on the exhale, this time falling all the way to the floor. The supporter needs to take special care not to be hurt while trying to support the mover.

7) As the mover becomes more comfortable with the falling movement, and more trusting of the supporting person, the mover may experiment with falling sideways, or even backwards. The supporter needs to be flexible in responding to the motions of the mover, perhaps falling with the mover, offering himself/herself as a pillow for landing.

8) When the mover has finished exploring falling with support, the partners trade places and the supporter becomes the mover and works on being supported.

IX. MOVING OUT: A DRAWING BECOMES A MOVING PICTURE.

Physical and emotional pain often occur when we unconsciously hold tension in our bodies. Try this remedy for discovering how and where you are holding tension and for experimenting with getting the energy to move on out. Anna Halprin calls this type of process psychokinetic visualizations. For this activity you will need to have some art supplies handy. Prepare to have a large newsprint pad and crayons or colored marking pens nearby.

1) After completing one of the exercises above or some other physical activity, lie down on the floor on your back.

2) Closing your eyes, imagine that you can send your awareness, like a search light, through the inside of your body.

3) Begin at the top of your head and travel down your body, sensing behind your eyes, inside your nose, inside your mouth. (If you have trouble doing this, swallow, and you will feel the inside of your throat.)

4) After you have completed sensing your entire body down to your feet, send the search light back up through your torso to the top of your head.

5) Now imagine what your body would look like from the inside, if you had a special camera that could view the inner terrain.

6) Sit up slowly, take art materials and draw your body from what you have sensed from the inside. Use color and texture to highlight areas that stand out to you. Indicate areas that you are not able to feel from the inside.

7) Fasten your drawing to a wall where you can view it without having to hold it.

8) Become your drawing, assuming the posture and angles represented.

9) After you have gotten a feel of your drawing as a still image, allow yourself to move so that you (as your drawing) become a moving picture. Name your picture if a title occurs to you at this point.

10) Go back to the still position and see if there is some other way that this picture (and your body) could move.

11) Return to your position on the floor and notice if your body feels any differently from when you began.

12) Ask yourself, "What does this picture say about my life?"

Transformation Of A Career: A Healing Ritual

The scene is a forested backyard. Folding chairs have been placed in rows facing a raised deck overlooking a small stream. Approximately 30 participants file into the backyard and are seated while the Shaker song, "Tis A Gift To Be Simple," plays in the background. The presiding woman minister begins.

"Dearly beloved, we are gathered here in the sight of God, the university, the county, nation, and world to witness and participate in the transformation of the career and life work of this woman, Sheila Collins. Since all members present have had ample and sufficient opportunity to object to this transformation, (committees having met, votes having been counted, petitions having been heard, pipes having been smoked, hands having been wrung, and floors having been paced), I hereby declare that all persons involved with this woman's career life must herein and after *forever hold their peace!*"

READING

An except from Jean Auel's *Clan of the Cave Bears* is read by Sheila's son, Kevin. Bringing in the archetypical element of shunning, Kevin reads of how Ayla, girl of the Clan, is banished for using a weapon (a sling shot) which is against the traditions of the Clan.

"The clan didn't care if the spirit took the body with it, or left the unmoving shell behind, but they wanted the spirit of Ayla to go, and go quickly."

DISTRIBUTION OF THE ELEMENTS

(A filing cabinet on a dolly is wheeled from the building at this point, accompanied by pall bearers, colleagues and dignitaries from Sheila's past career life.) The minister continues: "It is important that we remember that the contents of this cabinet, though containing all of the original manuscripts written by Dr. Collins prior to and during her academic career, including articles (published, rejected and under editorial consideration at this time), book chapters, course syllabi for both credit and non-credit courses, grant proposals (funded, rejected and under editorial consideration at this time), and all memos and letters, carbons of memos and letters, and later, xerox copies of memos and letters. In spite of the breadth and depth of the material which we are about to throw into this fire, we must remember that the real abilities, gifts, visions, and spirit of their author remain ever with us. These items, though they represent thousands of hours of effort, dedication, discipline, uncooked meals, sleepless nights, and missed television programs (not to mention missed ski trips, missed sporting events, missed soap operas and ladies' luncheons), — these items do not represent the real creativity, artistry, scholarship, and acquired "street smarts" that the woman, Sheila Collins, has developed during this period of her career/life work." (As the song "All My Life's A Circle" is played, the head pall bearer opens the first drawer of the file cabinet and distributes the contents to individuals in the audience.)

TESTIMONIALS

When all the manila folders had been distributed, the minister said, "We now take time to share our reflections, feelings, visions, and versions of Sheila Collins' work life." Friends, colleagues, former students, and family members remembered aloud aspects of Sheila's career life. Mention was made of her free spirit, creativity, and of her tendency to be "ahead of her time."

ELEVATION

The minister directs the congregation: "Please stand, raise your manila folders and envelopes to the heavens and repeat after me: We offer these gifts to the Great Mother as evidence of our faith in the strength of her spirit, that same spirit which is reflected in these writings and other creative expressions of author, Sheila Collins. In spite of the lack of evidence of appreciation, reward, recognition, monetary compensations, the granting of tenure or the real and authentic opportunity to earn same, we hereby affirm our belief that the Great Mother will see to the success and fulfillment of all those who have attempted to serve her. We affirm our belief that the Great Mother will insist that these offerings of Dr. Collins and those of her courageous co-authors and collaborators will not be burned in vain. Neither will she set in motion a vengeful spirit, since she alone fully appreciates the progress having been made since ancestral sisters were personally burned at other stakes of institutional righteousness. Amen. Praise God and prepare to fuel the fire."

READING

Sheila's husband, Richard, selected and read the story of the origin of the pipe from *Black Elk Speaks*. He told of two scouts seeing a woman approaching, and one of them was foolish and had bad thoughts of the woman. When he approached her a cloud came and covered them, and when the cloud was gone, the man was a skeleton covered with worms. The story continues as the woman went into a teepee singing:

> *With visible breath I am walking.*
> A voice I am sending as I walk.
> In a sacred manner I am walking.
> In a sacred manner I walk."

OFFERING

(People in the congregation begin a procession around an incinerator and each person, in turn, throws the folder he or she is holding into the fire. The song, "It's In Everyone Of Us," plays in the background. Meanwhile, a singer chants in a minor key the curriculum vitae of Dr. Collins, gradually increasing the tempo until a drummer joins in, syncopating the rhythm. The congregation snaps fingers to the beat.)

READING

A passage from the poem, *"Burnt Norton,"* by T.S. Eliot, was read by Sheila's son, Ken.

Improvisation/Transformation

The song, "Lord of the Dance," is sung by Sheila's daughter, Corinne, in accompaniment to her mother's improvisational dance.

CELEBRATION

As the solo dance ends, Sheila leads the ritual participants in a community dance which is accompanied by "The Song of the Soul." A reception follows the ceremony.

References

Auel, Jean M.,*The Clan Of The Cave Bear* (Bantam Books: New York, 1985), p.271.

Neihardt, John G., *Black Elk Speaks* (University of Nebraska Press, Lincoln, Nebraska, 1981), p.5.

APPENDIX D

A SPECIAL RESOURCE

After sending a written request for permission to use a few lines from the song, "Let There Be Peace On Earth," I received a phone call from Jill Jackson Miller, the woman who, with her husband, wrote the song in 1955. After finding out more about the book I was writing, Ms. Miller generously suggested that I include all the words to her song. As she told me some of the stories about the song and how it has been used throughout the years, we both agreed it was a valuable resource for the readers of this book. It is offered here as a gift from the song's author, who believes as I do that caregivers must take care of themselves as well as taking care of others.

Let there be peace on earth,
And let it begin with me.
Let there be peace on earth,
The peace that was meant to be.

With God our creator,
Children all are we,
Let us walk with each other
In perfect harmony.

Let peace begin with me,
Let this be the moment now.
With every step I take
Let this be my solomn vow,

To take each moment and
Live each moment in peace eternally.
Let there be peace on earth
And let it begin with me.

(original, "with God as our father, brothers all are we. Let me walk with my brother...".)

© 1955 by Jan-Lee Music, c. renewed 1983. Used by permission of Jill Jackson Miller, Jan-Lee Music.

APPENDIX E

BODY-ORIENTED RESOURCES

A major theme of this book has been that taking care of oneself involves taking care of one's body. Attending to the needs of the physical body provides access and benefit to the mental, emotional, and spiritual dimensions of the self as well. Throughout this book references have been made to "body-work," "movement work," and "body-oriented psychotherapy." The following resource guide is offered to assist you in selecting the methods and systems that are right for you in particular phases of your selfcaring, selfhealing journey.

PHYSICAL

All bodywork systems deal with the physical body, but the ones listed below focus primarily on structure, alignment, posture, and the mechanical functioning of the body.

Massage Therapy - Most people's view of what constitutes massage is much more narrow than the repertoire of a well-trained and experienced massage therapist. Swedish message, which involves long smooth strokes for a sense of connection between areas of the body and light strokes to facilitate relaxation, fits most people's view of massage. Sports massage, which is a deep tissue massage to relieve sore muscles is another popular style of massage. But experienced massage therapists are likely to include many techniques in their work, developing their own synthesis of styles, perhaps including some of the techniques listed below. Contact American Massage Therapy Association for therapist referral or curriculum approved schools. 1130 W. North Shore Ave., Chicago, IL, 60626, (312) 761-AMTA.

Alexander Technique - Named after its founder, F.M. Alexander, an Australian actor, this system aims to assist people in changing the way they use themselves physically as they perform everyday tasks. Alexander teachers work one-on-one with students, offering suggestions primarily through gentle touch and minimal verbal instruction. The technique seeks to reduce effort, restore neuromuscular balance, and increase self-awareness. The method is well known in England, and John Dewey and Aldous Huxley were enthusiastic supporters. For information regarding qualified practitioners contact Lena and Michael Frederick, P.O. Box 408, Ojai, CA, 93023 (805) 646-8902.

Feldenkrais Method - Developed by Israeli physicist Moshe Feldenkrais, this work has two components, Awareness Through Movement (a form of exercise done slowly in groups) and Functional Integration (a practitioner does hands-on gentle manipulation which increases awareness while inhibiting habitual movement patterns). For a list of qualified practitioners contact The Feldenkrais Guild, 1776 Union Street, San Francisco, CA, 94123, (415) 776-1776.

Rolfing - Named after founder Ida Rolf, this system involves a series of 10 sessions of deep tissue manipulation, each involving different areas of the body. The goal is to free the body from chronic tension for increased range of motion and improved posture. Contact The Rolf Institute, P.O. Box 1868, Boulder, CO, 80306, (303) 449-5903.

Chiropractic - The Doctor of Chiropractic specializes in the neurological and structural relationships of the body and their effect on health and disease. Hands-on manipulation is used to realign the body and to allow organs to function properly. Contact American Chiropractic Association, 1701 Clarendon Blvd., Arlington, VA 22209, (202) 276-8800.

Osteopathy - Osteopathic physicians are medical doctors, many of whom perform a gentle hands-on manipulative treatment to align the body and assist the recuperative system of the body. One practitioner, John Upledger, has taken this work further and has trained massage therapists, physical therapists and others to use his method, CranioSacral Therapy. One aspect which he calls Somato-Emotional Release deals with the emotional connections to the physical imbalances. Contact Upledger Institute, 11211 Prosperity Farms Road, Palm Beach Gardens, Florida, 33410, (407) 622-4334. For osteopathic physicans contact American Osteopathic Association, 142 E. Ontario, Chicago, IL (312) 280-5800.

Acupuncture or Acupressure(Shiatsu)- Acupuncture is the technique (from Chinese medicine) of inserting fine metal needles into the skin to treat ailments and relieve pain. Acupressure uses the same 100 to 150 pressure points but substitutes finger pressure for the needles. Can be used for prevention of illness and as an aid in childbirth and surgery. Contact Accupressure Institute, 1533 Shattuck Ave. Berkeley, CA. 94709, (415) 845-1059. or American Shiatsu Association, 295 Huntington Ave., Boston, MA. 02015, (617) 236-2286.

EMOTIONAL

Some body work systems engage in physical activities or movements primarily to evoke an emotional response. By expressing the unexpressed, the energy the person has been using to inhibit is freed for more productive endeavors.

Reichian - Wilhelm Reich, a student of Freud's, placed the body in a central role in personality theory. He developed a technique to mobilize feelings through breathing and hands-on contact and pressure aimed at dissolving what he called "character armour" in the body. One of the most direct line developments from Reich's work in this country is the following:

Bioenergetics Therapy - Designed by Alexander Lowen, this system engages clients in breathing activities and postures which stress the body to the point of emotional release. This system emphasizes the importance of sexual expression and release. The practitioner assists the client in connecting the physical tension and emotional release with the issues and situations from their past and present life experience. Contact The Institute For Bioenergetic Analysis, 144 East 36th Street, New York, NY 10016, (212) 532- 7742.

Lomi Bodywork - A connective tissue therapy and psychotherapy, Lomi was created by a physician, Robert Hall, and Richard Heckler, a psychologist, in the early 70's. Gestalt Therapy is a part of the verbal aspect of this integrative approach, along with hands-on touch. The practitioner directs the client 's attention to muscular tension so they may discover *how* they are *who* they are. Contact Lomi School Training, 4101 Middle Two Rock Rd. Petaluma, CA. 94952 (707) 778-6505.

MENTAL-(INTEGRATIVE)

The systems in this section are integrative, using the body to access physical, mental, emotional, and spiritual aspects of the person, and to assist the person in integrating these dimensions of the self.

Rubenfeld Synergy Method - Developed by Ilana Rubenfeld, this method is a synthesis of Gestalt Therapy, Feldenkrais, and Alexander work to which imagery, hypnosis, and the use of humor have been added. Through gentle touch and movement, clients are encouraged to discover the connection between their physical tensions and the issues and feelings of their past and present life. Contact Rubenfeld Center, 115 Waverly Place, New York, NY, 10011, (212) 254- 5100.

Hellerwork - Developed by Joseph Heller, a former Rolfer, this method consists of at least 10 sessions, working on movement of the structure of the body to restore natural balance. The client is encouraged to explore the feelings and images which arise as the practitioner works with the deep tissues of the body. Contact Hellerwork, 514 4th Street, San Raphael CA, 94901, (415) 456-5533.

Hakomi Method - Developed by Ron Kurtz, Hakomi is a body-centered psychotherapy that works with the principles of nonviolence and mindful- ness. The practitioner approaches the client with gentle respect and supports the person's accessing of core memories. By physically taking over the client's chronic holding patterns, the client has the opportunity to let go of the tension and experience whatever feelings or memories the holding is connected to. Pat Ogden with Ron Kurtz has developed a tablework or hands-on version of Hakomi which includes verbal instruction. Contact The Hakomi Institute, 2017 B 10th Street, PO Box 1873, Boulder, CO, 80306, (303) 443-6209

Movement and Expressive Arts Therapy - An integrative way of working with dance, drama, visual arts, and music is the work done by Anna Halprin and her associates at Tamalpa Institute. A psychokinetic visualization process is used to move back and forth between movement, felt sensation, imagery, and symbols and drawing. Core material is often generated, explored, and expressed. Dr. Halprin's work goes beyond therapy of the individual to include a collective creativity process and community transformation through events such as the annual Circle The Earth Peace Ritual. Contact Tamalpa Institute, P.O. Box 794, Kentfield, CA, 94914, (415) 461- 9479.

Trager Work - Designed by physician Milton Trager, Trager Work consists of a systematic set of gentle shaking, stretching, and rocking movements done while the person is lying on a table. The aim is to assist the client in letting go of tension, releasing and lengthening. Imagery and meditation are also used. There is also a dance form (Mentastics) abstracted from the table work which is used to maintain the balance gained. Contact The Trager Institute for Psychophysical Integration and Mentastics, 10 Old Mill, Mill Valley, CA, 94941, (415) 388-2688.

SPIRITUAL

Methods and traditions which use movement to attain a higher consciousness are listed here. These bodywork traditions often use the concept of energy as in the chakras, or energy centers. Practitioners of these methods may consider themselves transfering healing energy from themselves to another, or altering their own body/mind state to a state of oneness with all. Yoga, shamanism and faith healing would fall into this category of body work.

Therapeutic Touch - Developed by a nurse, Delores Krieger, this system has been taught to nurses and other health professionals around the United States. Practitioners place themselves in a meditative state but do not actually touch the patient. They touch only the energy field or aura around the person in order to stimulate the recuperative powers of the patient. For more information contact Dolores Krieger, 70 Shelly Ave., Port Chester, N Y, 10573.

Tai Chi - The oldest of the martial arts, this movement activity is called a "moving meditation." A person, alone or simultaniously with others, moves as effortlessly as possible through positions or postures expressing the notion that change is the only constant in the universe. Tai Chi Association, 2620 E. 18th St., Brooklyn, NY, 11235.

Polarity Therapy - Developed by Dr. Randolf Stone, this system involves manipulation, exercise, diet, love, and thought to promote relaxation and help maintain normal body functioning. Contact Polarity centers in Boston, 41 Dunster Road, Jamaica Plain, Massachusetts, 02130, (617) 522-8450 or 28779 Via Las Flores, Murrieta Hot Springs, CA, 92362, (714) 677-7411.

Yoga - There are many ancient and modern schools of yoga but one resource that fits the selfcaring, selfhealing theme of this book is the work of Eleanor Criswell Hanna. A Professor of Psychology, she is involved in yoga and the field of biofeedback. Dr. Hanna has worked closely with her late husband, Thomas Hanna in the development of the field of Somatics. She continues a journal by that name and a research institute. Contact Novato Institute, 1516 Grant Ave., Suite 212, Novato, CA, 94945.

INDEX

● ●

AFFIRMATIONS

EXERCISES

POEMS

ABOUT THE AUTHOR

Sheila K. Collins has been a dancing social worker for over twenty years. She has an M.S.W. from Wayne State University in Detroit, Michigan and a PhD from the University of Nebraska at Lincoln. Prior to her career as a professor in social work and her work as a psychotherapist, she was a professional dancer.

She has, among other things, been a member of a regional ballet company, toured with a national company of a Broadway show, and been assistant director of a modern dance company, dancing in churches and synagogues.

To her roles as a therapist, teacher, and writer, she brings her dancer's perspective of creative collaboration and a concern for the person performing the helping role. Through research and publications she has explored the realities of caregivers' work lives. To bring creative change to the large system level, she founded, with others, organizations such as the Center For Co-Equal Education in Nebraska and the Women and Work Research and Resource Center in Texas.

In addition to her work as a therapist and teacher, helping people to access the physical, feminine, and creative aspects of themselves, she presents workshops and training seminars for helping professionals and other caregivers on how to become more selfcaring and selfhealing. Currently she is co-director of Iatreia Institute For The Healing Arts, a wholistic mental health center in Fort Worth, Texas.